MARK PURDEY, born in 1953, turned down [...] start his own organic farm at the age of 19. [...] started to teach himself neurobiology and in th[...] worldwide field research to discover the truth behind BSE, CJD and other neurodegenerative diseases. He was a vociferous campaigner on these issues, making TV programmes, publishing articles in peer-reviewed journals and lecturing at many prestigious institutions. He died in November 2006 of a brain tumour and is survived by his wife and eight children.

NIGEL PURDEY was born in 1951 and attended the Universities of London and South Bank. He taught classical guitar for a number of years, and for the last 25 years has worked in architecture. He has had Chronic Fatigue Syndrome for 18 years and this spurred him to research its links with toxic exposure. He soon developed an interest in his brother's work and accompanied him on several research trips, making several short films of their journeys.

ANIMAL PHARM

ONE MAN'S STRUGGLE TO DISCOVER THE TRUTH
ABOUT MAD COW DISEASE AND VARIANT CJD

MARK PURDEY

EDITED BY NIGEL PURDEY

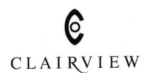

CLAIRVIEW

To the memory of Lionel Bateson Purdey
1886–1958

Clairview Books
Hillside House, The Square
Forest Row, East Sussex
RH18 5ES

www.clairviewbooks.com

Published by Clairview 2007

A catalogue record for this book is available from the British Library

ISBN 978 1 905570 11 9

Cover by Andrew Morgan Design
Typeset by DP Photosetting, Neath, West Glamorgan
Printed and bound by Cromwell Press Limited, Trowbridge, Wiltshire

Contents

Acknowledgements

I would like to thank the following for help in preparing this book —

Bob Woffinden and Brigid McConville for permission to draw on their articles 'The seeds of madness', *The Guardian Weekend*, 13 August 1994, and 'An expert in his field', *The Times Magazine*, 6 May 2000, respectively.

Margaret Purdey, Robb Bradstock and John Barkhausen for their personal recollections.

Jane Barribal for help with Mark's website articles.

Nigel Purdey

Foreword

by Bob Woffinden

'What a relief to breathe fresh clean air', commented Mark as we left my home in Hackney.

Even though I always knew to expect the unexpected with Mark, I was slightly taken aback. 'But, Mark,' I protested, 'this is grimy, run-down, inner-city London – and you live between the Quantock and the Brendon Hills in one of the most heart-stoppingly beautiful and unspoilt parts of the country.'

'You'd be surprised,' he replied. 'We get lots of chemicals and noxious fumes coming at us across the Bristol Channel from the heavy industry of south Wales.'

In every fibre of his body, it seemed, Mark was acutely sensitive to whatever was harmful in the environment. It was a sensitivity he'd developed after the life-changing experiences of watching a bird in a field keel over and die immediately after aerial pesticide-spraying, and then reading Rachel Carson's *Silent Spring*.

He soon realized that the natural world faced overwhelmingly powerful enemies, as the pharmaceutical companies looked to swell their profits by muscling in on agriculture. Within a few years, every aspect of farming would be dictated by the commercial interests of the multinational conglomerates. As Mark understood at a very early stage, this affected all of us profoundly. You could have your food with chemicals or without; though if you wanted it without, then, in a curious reversal of standard economic principles, you had to pay extra.

Mark entered the lists against the authorities on that day in 1984 when he was told he had to apply a pour-on insecticide to his cows or face the consequences of court action if he refused. He refused. No doubt the Ministry of Agriculture, Fisheries and Food (MAFF) anticipated a routine victory; but Mark was able to prove in court that, far from understanding the toxicological implications of their actions, the officials didn't even understand the legislation they thought they were enforcing. Round One to Mark.

That was his first conflict with the men and women from the Ministry, and it laid the foundation for his subsequent battles with authority. He would not accept blithe official reassurances or the platitudes of the professionals; and so began his lifelong campaign to find out what was doing precisely what damage to whom.

Pesticides may well kill the pests, but what else might they be doing? What other harm might they be inflicting – on the rest of the natural world, on those administering them, and on everyone else?

For years farmers routinely applied pesticides in haphazard ways – without basic precautions or protective clothing – that were condoned and even encouraged by manufacturers. There was a dreadful inevitability about what happened afterwards. Farmers and agricultural workers became victims of organophosphate poisoning – which, to compound their misfortune, was an illness the medical establishment was disinclined to recognize.

In those years, there were few to whom they could turn for assistance, but Mark was keenly interested in their plight. He was the one who was probing for details of what had happened, and trying to find ways of ameliorating their condition. His concern was entirely characteristic. He had an unquenchable generosity of spirit when it came to helping others, and a fierce intellectual curiosity when it came to resolving scientific mysteries.

Sadly, the general public never heard about the lives ruined by agricultural chemicals. The companies hired expensive lawyers and individual claims were strongly resisted. Given the potential for confounding factors that there is in everyday life (making it almost impossible to argue to standards of legal proof that substance X has caused condition Y), few could hope to succeed. In those cases where the circumstances were so overwhelming that claims did have to be met, the companies would settle out of court and attach a strict 'no publicity' clause. Claimants were always advised to accept.

This caused frustration and resentment among victims and those trying to act for them. The companies could keep the level of the awards low, as there was no recognized scale and no one knew what awards had been made in comparable circumstances. More importantly, the full scale of the problem would remain forever hidden. Indeed, the industry could even maintain the fiction that there were no problems at all. From his first-hand experience, Mark knew differently.

He wrote to me after I made a television documentary about the so-called Spanish 'cooking oil' disaster. In the film, I had pointed out that, significant as the incident had been (the toll was eventually put at over 1000 deaths and over 25,000 seriously injured, many of whom were permanently incapacitated; although those figures are certainly an underestimate), it had been misconstrued from the beginning. It may have been the most devastating food-poisoning in modern European history, but the supposedly contaminated cooking oil could not have been to blame. There were abundant reasons why not; it was, for example, as straightforward to find victims who'd never had the oil as it was to find whole areas of Spain where they'd used lorry-loads of the stuff without anyone suffering any ill-effects.

The overwhelmingly likely toxin was organophosphate pesticides on tomatoes grown under polythene tunnels. At just that point in time, organophosphate chemicals were being introduced to replace organochlorines (which had been discredited because Rachel Carson had exposed the damage they were doing) and were being shipped to agricultural businesses throughout the world. Had the truth about Spain come out, it would, of course, have been devastating for the industry. Yet the pharmaceutical companies managed to evade responsibility for the scandal and to protect their profits.

However, it has been necessary to sustain the myth. So, in the quarter-of-a-century since, research scientists worldwide have been engaged in the pointless task of trying to locate the toxin in the oil. Needless to say, they've never found it.

One's initial reaction to such a remarkable cover-up was that it could only occur in a country like Spain which at the time was a newly constituted democracy just emerging from almost 40 years of bleak authoritarian rule.

In retrospect, it was utterly naive to draw such a conclusion. We now know that such disinformation campaigns can be put into place anywhere, irrespective of how supposedly sophisticated societies are. In fact, the Spanish 'cooking oil' disaster became the template on which the chemical companies could construct future cover-ups – of which, of course, BSE became one of the most significant.

Mark's instinct had been sure. Dairy farmers had been coerced into subjecting their cattle to the physiological burden of having toxic chemicals poured along their backs. They then witnessed the spread of deadly disease amongst their herds.

Once again, an alternative culprit needed to be found. In Madrid, it had been the supposedly contaminated cooking oil; in England, it was supposedly contaminated meat and bone meal, the cattle feed. So the parallels with Spain began to accumulate. Mark attempted to point out some of the more obvious inconsistencies: that cows were developing the illness even though they had not even been born until after the supposedly infectious feed had been banned; on the other hand, no cattle in the countries to which the feed had been exported suffered any adverse reaction. Throughout the entire crisis, one blazingly obvious fact stood out: no home-reared cattle on fully converted organic farms ever developed BSE. It was simple: where there were no chemicals, there was no illness.

Nevertheless, the official theory had to prevail and outside voices had to be silenced. A crude Stalinist approach was adopted. Those who criticized the official orthodoxy were cruelly derided and dismissed as being 'unscientific' and lacking in objectivity. The reality, of course, was precisely the opposite: it was the official scientists who were being unscientific and who lacked objectivity.

If the feed manufacturers had indeed caused this terrible out-break then, naturally, one would have expected them to be prosecuted. However, in a repeat of what had happened when farmers suffered ill-health as a consequence of pesticide exposure, the industry and the ministry managed to ensure that these matters were determined behind closed doors and, most importantly, were not heard in open court. The hollowness of the Government's position would have been exposed had the matter reached court where searching questions would have been asked and the autho-rities would have been required to disclose relevant documents.

So, even though this ongoing tragedy must presumably have been caused by somebody, no one at all was prosecuted. By the time that there was a public inquiry under Lord Justice Phillips, much of the heat and nearly all of the newsworthiness of the issue had dissipated.

BSE, of course, led to the scares of CJD and other neurological diseases and uncertainty about precisely what was happening. At the outset, Mark had been airily dismissed as a harmless dilettante. Now, it seemed as though the scientific establishment needed to denigrate him more forcibly. My own thoughts about this were that if his theories were as cranky as the Ministry publicly asserted, then officials didn't have to worry about him; it was precisely because his theories were well-founded that they were alarmed and became more vituperative in their criticism of him.

Indeed, though never publicly admitted, the criticisms of Mark and others had hit home. In the aftermath of BSE and CJD, MAFF departed for the knacker's yard, its credibility in tatters. But the orthodoxy remained in place. Mark was still condemned for not being a proper scientist. The authorities would deprecate his work partly on the grounds that it was not being properly funded – in the full knowledge that they had done their darnedest to cut off all possible sources of funding for him.

Yet he was the one who had adopted a rigorous approach. He was the one who was ordering obscure papers from the British Library in the hope that they would enlighten his understanding of the various forms of the illnesses. He was the one who was actually going to the affected areas to do on-the-spot research.

It was Mark who, despite the overwhelming practical difficulties, was actively engaged with the issue. By contrast, the Establishment scientists, having checked that the industry grants had been paid into their accounts, could not have been less inquisitive.

I will remember so much about Mark, but what I will particularly remember is his charisma. As soon as you engaged in conversation with him, you knew you were in the company of someone very special. It is no surprise that so many were enthralled by him.

Now, his is a legacy that will endure. Indeed, one can predict with confidence that his influence will only grow over the coming decades. He had integrity and commitment and wit and vision and extraordinary intellectual energy, and all of us who knew him will never stop wishing he were still here.

London, September 2007

Preface

Mark had been preparing to write a book for several years but sadly died before he was able to do much work on the main text. He left a synopsis and it was clear from this that he was intending to redraft much of his older material, something he'd often done before when writing one-off articles. Although we didn't have any detailed discussions about the book, he said that if he didn't pull through the brain cancer he wanted me to complete it.

After Mark died, in November 2006, his publisher, Sevak Gulbekian, wanted to proceed with the project and we agreed the best way forward would be for me to work up Mark's existing material. I turned to a number of sources, such as his website, peer-reviewed articles, his BSE Inquiry statement, various articles by others about him and my own recollection of our discussions over the years.

I started from scratch on the Introduction, Afterword and Appendix. They're written in my own voice, apart from some personal contributions, including part of Mark's piece 'Tumerous Christmas' and material from newspaper articles by Bob Woffinden and Brigid McConville in the Appendix. I've shaped, edited and filled out Mark's chapters as I thought best, and the text is slightly coloured by my style.

I decided not to add numbered references to the text but instead listed some key papers and books for each chapter in the Principal Sources section. Anyone wanting precise references should look at Mark's papers relevant to the chapter and check out the references there. Many of these papers are available free on our websites: www.markpurdey.com and www.purdeyenvironment.com.

Mark and I both thought in very similar ways, so much so that often when we compared notes after some months apart we seemed to have travelled the same path, recognized the same problems and arrived at similar conclusions. I'd also worked pretty closely with him, making a series of films and accompanying him on trips to Iceland, Slovakia, Italy, Sardinia and around the UK. All this helped in the preparation of the book.

He worked on many other diseases throughout his life besides BSE and CJD (the transmissible spongiform encephalopathies – TSEs) such as bovine TB, multiple sclerosis, Machado-Joseph's and Guam syndrome. During the BSE years Mark was known as the 'organophosphate'(OP) man, but in fact he thought it was unlikely that the OP used to treat cattle for warble fly was the sole cause of BSE, but rather it precipitated the epidemic through various mechanisms involving copper homeostasis and oxidative stress.

Mark felt compelled to embark on his own research because the causal explanations of TSEs offered from official quarters continued to be unproven and implausible. If they'd proved their case or even produced a convincing argument he'd have shut up!

He went out into the field to study the diseases in their setting in life and set about decoding the environment where they were clustering. From his analysis he was then able to draw up his key theoretical statements, about the multifactorial causal interplay of munition contamination, ferrimagnetic crystal pathogens – manganese (and later barium, silver and strontium) – infrasound and oxidizing agents such as OPs and UV light.

He was the first person to come up with all of these points and although his work has not been fully proved there is strong evidence that oxidation and metal metabolism, in particular copper and manganese homeostasis, is the key to understanding TSEs. For example recent research has shown that manganese is able to cause the misfolding of the key prion protein into its abnormal form and also to give a positive result in a key test for prion disease known as the prionics test. (See Principal Sources and Further Reading section.)

Mark's research was limited in scope because it was largely funded by small donations from well-wishers and from his own pocket. He earned very little from any facet of his research work, including spin-offs such as lecturing and writing. Compare this with the position of the authorities, which have had millions of pounds of funding and have had every possible advantage in terms of facilities and scientific teams to make their case – one which still fails to demonstrate Koch's postulates after over 20 years of research.

It was a constant frustration to him that no journalist ever raised the key flaws in the official theories, listed at the end of Chapter 1, 'A Warble Fly in the Ointment', with any scientist or politician. No one in authority was ever challenged with these vitally important questions. Apart from some moving personal testimonies the scientific and political debate in the media on BSE and CJD has been indescribably anodyne and largely irrelevant.

Mark wanted the results of his work to be of real benefit to the world and there were usually simple practical strategies to benefit sufferers that flowed from it. For example, it is so obvious that what the Aborigines on the island of Groote Eylandt, described in Chapter 5, 'To the Ends of the Earth', need is help to reduce their manganese exposure. They don't need any more high tech research into their genetic profiles because it doesn't help them with their disease.

So often he found aspects of mainstream medicine to be stuck in the inertia of status quo and he desperately wanted to blast this apart so that useful, very often simple and non-trendy strategies could be introduced. This is not to say he was anti-science (when properly focused he had nothing but praise for high tech medicine). He was interested in the truth, and if an idea didn't stand up to scrutiny he jettisoned it and was fully aware of how one can easily slip into biased pathological scientific views.

At the end of his life he was confident of his theory but realized he needed to design and commission some studies to prove it. It's very sad that he didn't have a few more years to do this. Despite having a large grass-roots following I know he was frustrated that few people in positions of power had listened or responded to any of his findings; more often these people exploited him, which I suppose is the inevitable fate of the fundamentally decent guy.

I feel a tinge of sadness that he never got to see some of the more recent papers that support his position. He was the first person to come up with so many of these ideas and the first person to place them in the public arena, and my fear now is that if he's proved right he will not be credited. I hope that this book goes some way to put his vast contribution on record. He was a very creative and original thinker and when I was with him ideas just flowed from him constantly. I found him inspirational to work with and he taught me a huge amount. We'll all miss him enormously.

Nigel Purdey
London, April 2007

Introduction

Rebel with a cause

by Nigel Purdey

It was Christmas Day in 1953. I was two and a half years old and standing outside an ivy clad, pebbledashed nursing home in Broxbourne, holding hands with grandpa. Mum had got a very big tummy lately and she was inside having something done about it. Grandpa explained that I would soon have a brother or sister, but I wasn't interested and just wanted to be at home watching indoor fireworks and playing with my new train set. Next day mum came home with a small bundle of kicking, crying flesh, with a willy, and he was called Mark. I thought, perhaps this could be fun.

Mark and I grew up in a well-to-do household. Dad was a company director in the rubber business and a chartered accountant, but in his youth he'd been a semi-pro jazz pianist and had written comedy scripts to earn a living. Mum taught class music in the local primary school and was 100 per cent classical in her musical being, whilst dad was 100 per cent jazz.

On Saturday mornings dad would sit at our Boesendorfer baby grand in the hall and play a Count Basie style blues. He mumbled a lyric and beat out a wicked stride bass that drove relentlessly through the house, and vamped till mum was ready to go shopping; it was always a long blues. I would say Mark inherited the jazz gene from him and if this gene was at the root of his lateral creativity, then it was leavened slightly by mum's more sanguine genes.

Our parents were strict, quite formal and keen for us to learn etiquette, elocution and to mix in the right social circles. They'd met at a tennis club and were both very good players. Unfortunately we didn't inherit their interest in tennis, and this was a disappointment for them. One year dad made it to Wimbledon, although like many things in his past he never spoke of it.

Our great-great-grandfather was James Purdey, founder of the Purdey shot gun dynasty and a man of considerable determination and perfectionism. Looking at the old family photos and drawings from Victorian and Edwardian times our ancestors belonged to the hunting, shooting and fishing set and often rubbed shoulders with aristocracy.

Mark wanted this book to be dedicated to our grandfather, Lionel Purdey, who was a bit of a rebel and didn't go to work in the family gun business. We think that he signed up as a private in the Army and served in the First World War until he got shell shocked in 1916. He campaigned to get shell shock recognized and it appears that he was sectioned shortly after this, into the Springfield Hospital in Tooting, South London, where he tragically remained until his death nearly 40 years later.

At the time his wife was trying to set up as a Royal dressmaker and designer, and she eventually opened a successful shop in Sloane Street called 'Madam Eileen'. In his youth Lionel had been quite awkward, and what with his shell shock and campaigning it seems that his wife considered he was too difficult to handle and a liability to her career prospects, and this may have influenced the hospital admission.

I can't be sure that Lionel didn't need or benefit from hospitalization but once at Springfield he seems to have been totally cut off from his family and friends, because he was considered an embarrassment.

He was never spoken about in our house and we didn't even know we had a paternal grandad, until one day in late 1958 dad brought a small collection of personal effects – some socks, a razor and a hairbrush – into the bedroom and put them in his walk-in cupboard. Mum said something about them belonging to our late grandfather and it was left at that.

It was a chilling and pathetic image because this was Lionel, contained in these few personal effects, summarized in a few hospital notes — someone who would never really be part of anyone's personal memory. His existence in the later part of his life was effectively wiped of real relationships.

A few years ago, in one of those curious quirks of fate, whilst Mark was in the US lecturing, he happened to meet a woman who had come across an old photo of Lionel as a young man taken on a farm in Kansas. She'd been particularly struck by his charismatic looks and had researched the picture. She found out that Lionel was part of the Purdey gun family and had been a shell shock campaigner. After spending years trying to piece together his life story, one day his grandson Mark appeared. She then found out the tragic end to the tale, but at the same time she must have found some resolution to her quest to understand Lional's life through the chance meeting with Mark.

We grew up in the Hertfordshire village of Much Hadham, in a large listed house, which was neat and well decorated and had a big enticing garden. From an early age we explored its nooks and crannies and built camps and tree houses. In the fields beyond we played in the streams and charted new domains in the farmland that stretched for miles.

We were both sent at the age of eight to a boarding school called Forres in Swanage, nearly 200 hundred miles away from home. It was a tough place, and I remember it as always grey, with harsh pebbledashed elevations, battered by the sea winds and perched on a hill in that grey stone town. I rather like Swanage today.

Some of the teachers had a neat way with sadism; sensitive children like us found it hard to survive. The headmaster's technique for the extraction of mathematical answers was by a twelve-inch wooden ruler, which he'd beat progressively harder behind our left knee as we stood beside his desk. If you fumbled over an answer you would see his right hand slowly manoeuvring into the beating position — he'd deliberately draw out the foreplay, taking aim slowly, so that you would suffer all the more. And then thwack!

— the familiar sound of wood on flesh in English boarding schools. His strategy was to instil fear, as if by doing this he would somehow enable you to calculate the correct answer more quickly. Of course it had the opposite effect; you got progressively more flustered as the frequency and intensity of the beat increased. But when I looked into his weather-beaten and humourless face after he was done, I just saw the despair of an isolated and frustrated bachelor.

Children in those days had no power to question or complain, and our sense of injustice just turned inward and festered behind a closed mouth. Mark and I both developed contempt for this type of system. These early experiences led us to have a deep distrust not only of formal education but also of authority in general. We both naturally found an affinity with auto-didaction.

In the attic storey of the school there was one magical room where we were allowed to pursue hobbies, such as art and natural history. Here we could escape and discover treasures in abundance. We found the musty collections of beautiful mottled bird's eggs, and moths and then the butterflies, delicately crucified, with wings like miniature abstract expressionist diptychs, pinned in shallow mahogany drawers — quite unacceptable to today's sensibilities, of course.

Mark's interest in the natural world began here, and at about the age of ten he started bird watching and collecting eggs, butterflies and fossils. He channelled his passion into natural history, which offered him an imaginative foundation as well as a value system he could trust, in contrast to the cold regime of school. He inspired our father, who gradually developed into an obsessive bird watcher and bird photographer himself.

On Sunday afternoons at school we had another release in the form of walks in which we explored much of the brooding land-scape around the Isle of Purbeck — Ballard Down, the Tilly Whim caves, Chapman's Pool, the Jurassic coast, Durdle Door and Corfe Castle. They were all to seed in our imagination a deep love of landscape.

At home the collection of specimens grew steadily and Mark eventually took over most of our bedroom with a museum, centred on a three and a half metre long mahogany glass shop display case, which we bought in a junk shop in Westmill. It was soon filled with fossils – a huge ammonite, which is still in our garden to this day, geological samples, and assorted goodies such as sharks' teeth, animal skulls, bones and birds' eggs.

But an incident around this time was to have a deep impact on Mark. One summer day when he was watching birds in the fields beyond our garden he'd seen a plane spraying pesticides on the wheat fields. He later recalled: 'Soon afterwards I saw a blackbird quivering and dying at the edge of the field. That image affected me deeply and still haunts me today. It raised many questions in my mind about why this spraying was going on and what was it really doing to the environment.'

We both went on to a local public school called Haileybury and Imperial Service College. It was the sixties and things were loosening up in the real world outside, but public school lagged behind. 'It was all very militaristic and archaic,' Mark recalls. 'My education led me to question authority.' One of his school friends, Robb Bradstock, gave me his recollections of this time.

My first memory of Mark is from when I was 13. We both sat next to each other in the same class, taught by my father, and for some reason Mark used to stir things up by declaiming the names of rock bands – 'Jethro Tull! Ten Years After!' No one in the class knew who was doing it and I really relished this bravado, although it was embarrassing when he did it in my father's class. Mark was just totally driven to subvert things. In RE he was more cooperative and wrote amazing essays on the philosophical questions posed by aspects of religion, which really impressed my father, who used to comment, 'Where *does* he get it from?'

I had considerable family problems and left school at 16, but Mark and I kept in touch. He was always breaking out of school at nights and he would hitch or walk to meet me in the Golden Lion pub in Hoddesdon. We would drink illicit beer (not to excess) and talk of setting the world to rights. We were aware of issues such as pollution and the environment, but few people seemed to take any notice. There was still plenty of fresh air and not too much carbon dioxide about in those days.

At closing time we would sometimes move on to the woods near my home and light a bonfire and sit around till the early hours playing music, talking and drinking. Mark would then have to sneak back the three miles to school, but somehow he never seemed to get caught.

We also met up for the classic Sunday rock concerts at the Roundhouse in London and saw bands such as Ten Years After and Fotheringay, before they were well known. One night after a concert we missed the last bus and had to sleep in an open garage in a Camden back street. Mark, who used to take his sax and flute with him everywhere in those days, used his sax case as a very hard pillow! My home life was awful at this period and, after gaining some inspiration from reading *Down and Out in Paris and London* by George Orwell, I ran away from home. Mark had told me about a soup kitchen in the crypt of St Martin's in the Fields and I headed there. He became 'my spy' at Haileybury and after I'd been gone a couple of days he phoned to tell me that the police had interviewed him about my whereabouts. He assured me that, although put under extreme duress, even to the point of torture (he really liked to wind me up!) at the police station he hadn't cracked or divulged my address.

We often went travelling together with other friends and on one occasion after being chased by the police on a Cornish beach we somehow ended up in Bath, where Mark encouraged me to buy a clarinet in a junk shop. He taught it to me for a few months and we went on to form an eclectic folk/rock band called Lonely Air, which played songs Mark had written about Ireland.

He really seemed to understand how hard my childhood had

been and was very sympathetic and caring, which really made up for the horrible experiences at home. He had such a great sense of humour and would bring me out of my depression with his crazy stunts.

The summer after I'd left home he told me a lot about Ireland and being hooked I went over on the Cork ferry to meet him under the clock tower in Killarney, but he never made it. Later that year I visited him in Much Hadham and found he'd built a little sawdust kiln in the garden and was making very simple pots of clay from the bed of a local stream. This was my first experience of pottery and it inspired me to go on and study the craft and start my own pottery business near Macroom in the West of Ireland.

During our early teens we rediscovered the landscape experience we'd had at prep school. There was something about the meeting of history, colour, order and wildness in landscape that gave it a power to symbolize your inner being. It held up a penetrating mirror that showed you the deeper parts of yourself. It drew us in and hooked us.

One of the most memorable of those experiences was discovering the valley of the River Rib, about three miles across the fields behind our house.

On a baking July afternoon, just home from school, we walked off to the valley for the first time, following the footpath until we reached Barwick Ford. We then took the track to Latchford and strayed into an enticing wood just off the path. As we fought through the arches of dense trees we could just make out the ghostly shape of a building hunched into the bermed earth. It was like a simple croft cottage, but had thick concrete walls and had lost its roof years before. We couldn't imagine anyone living here and wondered what it was doing in the middle of a wood. The whole place had an uneasy but alluring silence. We pushed on through the interlocking arms of saplings, coming upon several more of the buildings and an unusual large concrete pool, which was choked with algae and buried under rampant branches. A grass snake splashed and writhed in the black water and swam away, disappearing into the undergrowth beyond. The darkness of the place was claustrophobic and we were relieved when we finally broke out into the fresh air of a magical sunlit glade. We returned there later that summer to wild camp and follow the gentle winding river below the wood. A few years later we discovered that the wood was the site of a gunpowder factory, which had been active during the Second World War.

Munitions seemed to form a leitmotif that connected various stages of Mark's life. Munition contamination was to emerge in his later research as the key to the way he understood the cause of several diseases.

Another munition incident from early childhood occurred when we were digging a pit in the garden and we'd unearthed an extraordinary cache of Second World War munitions. There were a couple of grenades, several rounds of 303 ammo and shell case. We cleaned them up and showed them off to Hadham's junior gangland culture. We were Godfathers after that, but within a few days dad discovered the armoury, the police were hastily called and our cache (and street cred) were removed.

A new outlet for Mark in his teens was music. Inspired by prog rock, folk and the new jazz of Soft Machine and John Surman, he taught himself the sax, flute and double bass. This led us to put on the Much Hadham Folk Festival for two years running in the back garden of the Red House, with all proceeds going to charity.

The first year was chaos – we made up a rickety stage from scrap planks and borrowed some rather dodgy PA equipment at the last minute, as Mark had forgotten to organize anything. We had also forgotten the mike stands and ended up improvising with a fishing rod, a broom handle and a bamboo cane and string. Unbelievably we also forgot to provide loos and drinks – luckily the Bull pub next door obliged on both counts.

In contrast the second year's festival was quite slick and professional. Gordon Giltrap headlined, with many excellent local acts in support and we had a rather good collection of PA equipment brought by the artists. The pub organized a drinks bar underneath the yew tree and we dug some primitive loos near the kitchen garden, astutely realizing that this juxtaposition could have some useful fertilizing implications.

Somehow our rather straight-laced parents coped (actually, I'm sure they secretly enjoyed it). Picture hordes of rather hippyish, stoned teenagers queuing up for the one downstairs loo in an impeccably furnished and decorated Georgian house. Well this is what mum and dad put up with. With around 250 people turning up, the garden heaved and, who knows, if we'd carried on for a few more years one of us might have become Hertfordshire's answer to Michael Eavis.

We spent several evocative family holidays in western Ireland at Inch and Castletownsend, where I endured a terrifying encounter with the ghost in the Castle guesthouse. Twenty-five years later I heard a radio documentary about the connection of the writers Somerville and Ross to Castletownsend and the castle, which they described as Ireland's most haunted place.

Mark fell in love with Ireland's unpretentious simplicity, its history and the natural power of the place. He came to admire much of the Celtic tradition from its music to the poetry of W.B. Yeats. During one of these holidays I remember he'd dragged us all along, on a wet day, to the Coosheen copper mine in County Cork, because he wanted to collect samples of copper ores. If I recall correctly, this was not a popular choice with the rest of the family; nevertheless he got his way. He disappeared for hours collecting rocks whilst we sat and had a picnic in the car park – British style. The mine was worked between 1840 and 1907 for various ores – cuprite, malachite and tetrahedrite. I believe it's now become a golf course.

As a result of this first foray into researching copper, we wrote a song together – Mark wrote the words and I wrote the music. The chorus went:

O they all came from Coosheen
A hundred years ago,
With a knowledge of mining
that green copper ore.

At about this time he started to become interested in ideas, particularly about the environment. He read Rachel Carson's *Silent Spring*, which galvanized him into his life's path. He wore John Lennon specs (which, like Lennon, he hated wearing), grew long flowing hair and generally cultivated a proudly scruffy, organic look.

He started developing the kitchen garden at the Red House as an experimental organic project. At the time we had a stalwart elderly gardener, called Walter Smith, who I don't think agreed with all of Mark's new-fangled organic gardening methods. Smith must have watched in disbelief at the young novice taking over and developing his kitchen garden. Most of the time Smith tactfully kept away, although we all knew he was itching to get stuck in and criticize Mark's methods. I think Smith was somewhat bemused as to why Mark had taken over the growing of the veg for the house when he was quite capable of doing it himself.

One night when Mark was climbing a wall to get back into school after one of his Hoddesdon all-night sessions he was caught by a master and promptly expelled.

After school he took a series of jobs, first labouring at a local plastics factory and then doing agricultural work in the Suffolk fens, where he lived in at an experimental farming and social commune. We also both did a stint as labourers at dad's rubber factory in St Albans.

Mark then moved away to another live-in job on a farm, which was in the process of converting to organic status, by the River Severn near Chepstow. During his time there he had to do some spraying with a pesticide which affected him badly. He went downhill quickly, becoming quite disorientated and withdrawn, and left the job.

He later turned down a place at Exeter University to read zoology and psychology. Instead he decided to set up an experimental organic farming community on the west coast of Eire. This didn't work out and he came back and settled in Pembrokeshire, where he married at 20, became an organic dairy farmer and had two children. The marriage broke up after three years, but he eventually settled down in the early eighties with a new partner Margaret, with whom he had six children and whom he married in 2006.

Mark's love of Ireland was to inspire him into improvising long bedtime stories for the children. He invented a cast of characters based on a mischievous young Irish girl called Mary O'Shea, her dog Holly Laws and their trusty sidekick, the Gannet, which had extraordinary magical powers. When I was there I often joined in by improvising different parts. The stories, which would often go on for hours, would verge on being small theatrical productions creating mayhem at bedtime. We definitely had as much fun as the kids did. He eventually wrote some of the stories down but never got round to getting them published.

Mark had a particular affinity with Jersey cows; he had started out with a single animal and gradually built up his herd. In the early days the growing family were squashed into a series of caravans, whilst the cows were put first and often seemed to have better accommodation than the family! In 1997 one of their cows achieved the highest recorded UK milk yield for the Jersey breed.

Besides milking Mark branched out into swede production, once spending a whole winter pulling the veg between milking. Every day he'd have to drive the swedes to Bristol, or sometimes London, in an ancient 30 cwt hired van. The rewards were not great in this business and when the axle on the van finally broke this provided a good excuse to stop.

The family had no car for several years; they used a tractor instead. Mark took Margaret to her first antenatal class on the back of his Leyland tractor. Margaret was so embarrassed by this she never went back again. The day she went into labour she drew the line at the tractor and insisted that Mark should borrow a car to get to hospital, but it broke down after only a few miles (they should have stuck with the tractor). Mark insisted on hitch-hiking the rest of the way, hoping that someone would take pity. They did.

By the 1980s their dairy farming business had become quite well established but a change in the law in 1982 led to a requirement in their area to use a powerful organophosphate pesticide to treat cattle for warble fly. This raised many issues for Mark as an organic farmer and he didn't trust the view of the Ministry of Agriculture that this pesticide was safe to use in the way it was decreed. A deadlock ensued between Mark and the Ministry, which ushered in the next chapter of his life.

1

A Warble Fly in the Ointment

In the mid-1980s, a novel neurodegenerative syndrome that became known as bovine spongiform encephalopathy (BSE) began appearing in cattle in the UK. The disease has annihilated thousands of cattle, as well as creating a fierce battleground between nations, vested interests, political parties, farmers, victim support groups and consumers. It was followed, in 1995, by the first case of the human equivalent of BSE, which became known as variant CJD. The shock waves of the BSE debacle have ricocheted around the world, reaching as far afield as Japan and North America.

BSE first struck at Pitsham Farm, near Midhurst, West Sussex in December 1984 and initially confounded the veterinary services. Two years later, and after a few hundred more cases, this condition was confirmed as a transmissible spongiform encephalopathy (TSE) similar to scrapie in sheep.

Despite the severity of the mad cow legacy, little attempt has been made to crack the causal riddle of the diseases, thereby leaving us with little insight into measures that would best treat, control and prevent this disease. The official hypothesis, which I've never seen fully set out in a peer reviewed journal, is that BSE is caused by various modes of exposure to brain material sourced from animals that have become contaminated by an infectious protein-only agent known as the prion – a malformed version of the normal prion protein that is found in all healthy mammalian brains and quite widely throughout the body.

The route of the supposed infection can be via abnormal prion contaminated feedingstuffs, injections of prion contaminated tissues (e.g. involving blood/growth hormone), cranial implantation with prion contaminated depth electrodes or merely through body to body contact (via saliva).

BSE was blamed by MAFF on the feeding of the rendered remains of scrapie-affected sheep to cattle. At that time both sheep and cattle remains were incorporated into meat and bone meal (MBM) cattle feed. The ruminant remains were used to boost the protein content of concentrated feeds and were a replacement for the more expensive arable crop proteins that can also be used. The Royal Society proposed a different version of this theory, to get around the crossing of the sheep to cow species barrier; they suggest a spontaneous mutation in the prion gene in a single cow caused the disease. BSE was subclinical at first and spread slowly throughout the UK, via MBM feed, and eventually became a full-blown epidemic. A feed ban was introduced in 1988 in the UK, to prevent ruminant protein being fed to ruminants; it was thought, incorrectly, that this would quickly eradicate the disease.

A relaxation in the temperature and manufacturing techniques of the MBM rendering process in the UK was blamed for enabling the scrapie agent to survive and then to affect cattle, producing BSE. The temperature was apparently lowered from 138 or 150°C (I've seen different figures quoted) to an unspecified temperature.

There was also a cessation in the rendering process in the use of solvent extractors, such as acetone, to recover the last scraps of meat.

But scientific evidence is being amassed which indicates that BSE and vCJD could both result from separate exposure of bovines and humans to the same cocktail of toxic environmental factors — copper lowering factors, metal microcrystals and low-frequency sonic shock — and not from the ingestion of the one species by the other.

The story of BSE began for me back in 1984 when I was a dairy farmer at Halse, near Taunton. I had a herd of 80 pedigree Jerseys and my practice had been to use an organic pesticide, derris powder, to control warble fly when necessary. Derris was on

MAFF's approved list until 1982 and is a naturally occurring compound, which I'd used successfully in the past to treat warble fly. The larvae of the fly burrow in through the cow's hide and live within the body of the cow, usually damaging both the meat and the hides. Milk yield can be reduced by as much as 25% and therefore this humble fly has considerable economic consequences for both dairy farmers and the leather industry.

In 1982 measures were passed that enforced a twice annual application of a uniquely concentrated dose (20 mg/kg body weight) of a systemic acting organophosphate (OP) insecticide called phosmet for the control of warbles on UK cattle. Britain was the only country to prescribe this treatment at this concentration, twice yearly, regardless of the fact that when it was administered many of the cows, as either spring or autumn calvers, would be in the early stages of pregnancy when the embryo is most vulnerable. Moreover, the cow as a species was especially vulnerable to OPs, having a low level of the nerve protecting enzyme cholinesterase, which OPs specifically target.

Studies had also indicated there was a chance that OP residues could contaminate cows' milk after treatment and I was concerned that this might cause long-term delayed neurotoxic damage to susceptible types of cows and humans.

Many cattle would also have been undergoing treatment with phosmet lice treatments, fly repellents or worm drenches as well as the warblecide, and this could exacerbate any latent problems. I feared that there would be an epidemic of some kind of neuro-degenerative disease as a legacy of the warble fly treatment.

I was also concerned for the welfare of my partner, Margaret, who was then pregnant, as there had been cases where farmers' wives had miscarried after coming into contact with OPs. I was also aware of a variety of other adverse health effects strongly associated with OPs, which I was witnessing in my rural community and dis-covering in my early research.

As I expected the Ministry didn't accept my arguments and, as my cattle were not treated with phosmet, they imposed restrictions on my livestock and threatened prosecution. I wrote several letters to, among others the Prime Minister, the Minister of Agriculture, MPs, MAFF's Advisory Service (ADAS), the District Veterinary Officer at Taunton (DVO), the Central Veterinary Laboratory (CVL) and the Health and Safety Executive. The Ministry however didn't change their position and they informed me that they intended to treat my cattle and to recover their expenses from me. I had no option but to take legal action and challenge the 1982 Order by an application for judicial review.

I had the support of Dr Alastair Hay, of the Department of Chemical Pathology, Leeds University. My lawyers sought an order quashing the Minister's Enforcement Notice and argued that the Ministry had been acting unlawfully by enforcing a pour-on treatment with OPs. They had no powers to make the 1982 Order under the Diseases of Animals Act 1950, which only empowered the Minister to enforce treatment with a vaccine or a serum.

On 27 March 1985 Mr Justice Woolf granted me leave to apply for judicial review. At the hearing we reached an agreement that my dairy herd would be exempted from the OP treatment. I accepted a compromise in which my heifers had to be treated with an alternative pesticide – ivermectin, a non-OP, which nevertheless makes cows' milk unfit for human consumption for 28 days.

As time went on I became increasingly interested in the general health effects of OPs, and in 1987 I submitted evidence to the House of Commons Agriculture Committee inquiry into the effects of pesticides into human health. I linked OPs with brain disorders such as multiple sclerosis, Parkinson's and Alzheimer's disease. I also authored and presented my first TV documentary on the subject for BBC2, called *Aggrochemicals*. After the programme I was inundated with letters and calls from people who thought that their unusual illnesses were caused by exposure to pesticides and other toxic compounds.

In October 1987 I clashed with the authorities over an article by

Dr Gerald Wells, which was published in the *Veterinary Record*. I was incensed by the casual way in which some of the research I'd referenced was dismissed. I wrote to *Farmers Weekly* in December 1987 querying why the journal had dubbed my postulated link-up between phosmet exposure and BSE as 'ill-informed rumour mongering'. I said: 'My own independent survey on some of the farms inflicted with this crippling neurotoxicity have revealed that phosmet treatment and a brand of feeding stuff compounded from insecticide-treated raw materials are the common denominators on these farms.'

I also pointed out in my letter that two researchers, Drs Cavanagh and Bouldin, had observed 'intraneuronal ballooning vacuoles' and 'neurofibrillary proteinaceous conglomerations' in the grey matter of the brain stem in nerve tissue of animals poisoned by OPs. These features resemble major aspects of BSE pathology.

It was in the summer of 1991 that BSE struck first on my new dairy farm in Elworthy, Somerset. One of my cows, Churnside Birthday, which I'd bought in from a chemically run farm, had developed a 'staggers' disorder, which my vets thought was probably BSE. I raised with the Chief Veterinary Officer the possibility that exposure to OPs was upsetting the cow's neuro-psychiatric equilibrium and pointed out a publication where OPs had been shown to induce spongiform encephalopathy in three victims. My points were rejected, and the cow was slaughtered and BSE confirmed.

By this time I was starting to formulate a theory on BSE, and early in 1992 the *Ecologist* magazine published my first peer-reviewed article which drew links between BSE and phosmet usage. I argued that there was a growing body of evidence that OP insecticides could play a key role in the development of BSE. The epidemic was worst in areas designated by MAFF as warble fly eradication zones throughout the 1980s. Voluntary treatment of cows with phosmet was urged by MAFF in areas outside the compulsory zones. I had noticed that there was no record of any cow born and raised on an organic farm dying of BSE. The great majority of organic farms had avoided using the high dose type of OP and it is interesting that many cows on those farms may have been fed the bonemeal concentrates blamed for the disease. I had also spoken to dairy farmers who had BSE in their herds and who had never used the incriminated MBM feed on their farm.

I listed similarities between BSE and chronic low dose OP poisoning and suggested that it might also 'switch on' replication of the abnormal prion protein that was supposed to cause BSE. The *Western Gazette* of 19 March 1992 reported Professor Lacey, who had been one of the peer-reviewers of my paper, as saying that 'it looks increasingly likely there may be one or more precipitating agents that trigger off BSE and it is possible that insecticides are involved'. He also later wrote that I had 'certainly produced strong evidence for a causal effect between exposure to [OP] chemicals and the precipitation of BSE-related symptoms'.

In the summer of 1992, Damson, another of my cows, which had been treated with an OP insecticide before I bought her, went down with BSE. I refused to hand her over for slaughter because I wanted to test my theory by trying an experimental treatment with an OP antidote. The DVO agreed that I could carry out the treatment and my vet, Christopher Budge, injected Damson with oxime and atropine sulphate, which are pharmaceuticals carried by troops in the Gulf War as an antidote to OP gas poisoning. The results were very exciting because within 90 minutes the cow appeared to have remitted and rose to its feet. Two days later, my vet and the vet from MAFF examined Damson but no more treatment was given. Over the following weekend Damson's condition deteriorated and I asked my vet to continue with the injections, which would be the normal protocol when treating OP poisoning. On the Monday the Ministry vet told me that Damson should be put down and Mr Budge said that he needed to take further advice before he could re-inject her. On the next day Damson collapsed. I wanted to go to the High Court to force the Ministry to let me continue the treatment, but the Ministry vet said that Damson had to be put down on welfare grounds. I was angry because there had been a very positive response to the OP antidote and it needed investigation.

Oximes are usually employed in acute cases of OP poisoning, often with atropine sulphate, and this was clearly not acute poisoning, but a Japanese Professor, Satoshi Ishikawa, had found benefits from this treatment in some chronic OP victims. I thought it was also possible that the positive effects of the treatment were coming from the atropine sulphate rather than the oxime. If there was no connection between the BSE condition and OP poisoning why did Damson respond so positively to what was a specific OP treatment? This result didn't prove that OPs caused BSE but science is about curiosity and the exploration of leads like this. I thought that someone wanted to avoid the embarrassment of the treatment working and the questions and inquiry that might flow from this. BSE was later confirmed in Damson on 20 August 1992.

My third case of BSE occurred in April 1993. It became apparent that Brainstorm had contracted BSE by vertical transmission from its mother, Churnside Birthday. Brainstorm hadn't eaten MBM or had phosmet treatment and she was born after the 1988 ban on using ruminant protein in feed for other ruminants. The animal was fed exclusively on organic feed and yet had all the signs of BSE. Its only link with the disease was that its mother had it.

The Government vet came on three occasions and observed typical BSE symptoms of myoclonus, nystagmus, tremors under the skin, hypersensitivity to touch and sound, fear of entering the milking parlour, weight loss and a vacant expression. I decided to start treating her with magnesium sulphate injections because I was also interested in the possible role of sulphates as an antidote to BSE. Within a few days of her first injection her symptoms had almost totally remitted. The government vet revisited my farm and said that in her view Brainstorm, although not totally healthy, no longer exhibited the symptoms of BSE and she withdrew the movement restrictions she had placed on my cow.

Brainstorm continued to live and milk on the farm until she was slaughtered in the conventional way in the autumn of 1996 and was then confirmed to have had BSE. Again I thought that this was a very significant result and needed more research. As usual it wasn't followed up by anyone.

I continued to write letters about my theory to, among others, my MP, Tom King, who became a supporter, and in April 1993 he wrote to John Gummer, the Minister of Agriculture. Mr Gummer reiterated the Ministry's unchanging view that 'detailed studies of the epidemic of BSE in cattle have not shown any connection between the use of such chemicals, either in a primary or con-tributory role, and the incidence of this disease. That this disease has been spread by the use of infected feed, the hypothesis on which the disease control policy is based, has been substantiated by analytical epidemiological studies and by the effects now seen on the incidence of disease in the younger age groups of cattle.'

I didn't accept this view at all because there was still no scientific trial that showed eating MBM produced BSE in any animal and there was growing contra evidence to the theory due to the absence of BSE in countries to which the feed was exported.

I gave a presentation at a special meeting with MAFF officials at the CVL on 17 January 1994. At the meeting they promised a longer look at my theory on OPs and BSE, but they ruled out scientists carrying out research into the theory, primarily due to costs to the taxpayer. We all agreed that the disease was slowly dying out, but the officials said this was because the scrapie contaminated food was banned in 1988. I didn't think this fitted because the rate of dying out was much slower than they had predicted, indeed we still have BSE occurring in 2006, and MBM hadn't caused BSE abroad. I said that I thought it was because particular pesticides were with-drawn or naturally phased out (e.g. the virtual eradication of the warble fly) at the end of the 1980s.

I kept badgering MAFF with my OP research and wrote to Mr Wilesmith at MAFF in December 1994, referring to a supportive letter from Professor Satoshi Ishikawa of Kitasato University. Professor Ishikawa, who is an expert on OP poisoning, said that he felt that my 'description of mad cows and warble fly to organophosphate compounds is exactly true'. Mr Wilesmith argued that I was being misled on the pathology and suggested that it was strange that there hadn't been a plethora of papers describing the histopathological changes associated with the TSEs as similar to OP poisoning, chronic or otherwise. I thought that it was interesting that MAFF had now admitted the existence of chronic OP poisoning, a phenomenon that they had already dismissed as illusory beforehand. I wasn't surprised that they were trying to break down Professor Ishikawa's pathological correlation between specific neurons which are vacuolated in OP chronic poisoning and the same neurons which Dr Wells cited as vacuolated in the first paper on BSE pathology.

An independent television company, Lauderdale Productions, was contracted by Channel 4 to make a documentary in the *Frontline* series about the OP perspective related to BSE and my work. They contacted Dr David Ray of the Medical Research Council (MRC) at Leicester, who'd invited me to lecture to his department at the University of Leicester. The TV company commissioned Dr Ray to test my theory experimentally. He was aware that it centred on the OP phosmet, nevertheless the TV company and the MRC agreed to use an alternative OP, called DFP, which was conveniently available. DFP is a markedly different type of OP to phosmet, and is not used on farms. Reluctantly I agreed to the compromise but on the basis that the oxone metabolite of DFP, which is also common to phosmet, was used.

As the results of the tests were kept secret from me, so that the film would contain a surprise element, I was annoyed to eventually learn that the oxone metabolite had never been used. I was aware from the start that recombinant prion protein without a glycolipid anchor was used and was concerned that this weakened the trial because the anchor could play a role in any interaction between

OPs and the prion. When the MRC received the results, they dis-regarded a minute amount of dose proportional binding of DFP to the prion as mere contamination of the protein with an impurity.

When Channel 4 came to pay for this work, I understand that the MRC replied that the work had already been paid for. They didn't say who had paid, but they did say 'MAFF owned the work'. I was disappointed with the trial because it hadn't tested my ideas at all. Nevertheless it did make me more resolved to fund a more sophisticated trial using phosmet and cell cultures. I took some heart because the reviews of the documentary were very good: Peter Paterson wrote in the *Daily Mail*, 'may be one of the most important documentaries transmitted in years'.

In 1996 I was summoned to see the EU farm commissioner, Franz Fischler, but made no headway with him. He said that because my work wasn't peer-reviewed he couldn't take it any further. But it was peer-reviewed. This was just appeasement.

Prior to February 1997, Lord Lucas, the MAFF spokesman in the House of Lords, gave a written answer to a question from Lord Lester in which he said that the Government had asked SEAC to re-examine my theory. He also indicated that the Government was aware of the new research by Dr Stephen Whatley, of the Institute of Psychiatry, into the effects of phosmet on prion protein cell cultures. This research was commissioned by myself and co-funded by myself and well-wishers. The results were eventually published in 1998 in the journal *Neuroreport*.

Dr Whatley exposed human neuroblastoma tissue culture cells to very low doses of phosmet, which interacted dramatically with the prion protein, causing it to traffic and to distribute abnormally in the cells. In the phosmet treated cells, three out of the four hitherto recognized abnormal characteristics specific to the TSE causing pathogenic prion were invoked. The alterations involved an increase in prion protein on the surface of the cells, an accumulation of prions in small organelles of the cell, and an abnormal resistance of the membrane anchored prion to cleavage by phospholipase C. These phosmet-induced reactions were specific to the prion protein and were proportional to the dose of phosmet introduced. The doses used were equivalent to what a cow would be likely to receive after warblecide treatment. This test failed to demonstrate protease resistance in phosmet-affected prions, but nevertheless the results were encouraging and suggested that some abnormal prion modification had been invoked by the introduction of phosmet.

I was invited to give a presentation at the 41st meeting of the Spongiform Encephalopathy Advisory Committee (SEAC) which was held on 15 April 1997. After the discussion SEAC asked two members, Professors Sir Colin Berry and Ian Shaw, to assess my theory on paper. On the basis of their findings, SEAC would decide whether to advise the Government to fund research into my theory. I was concerned that Professors Berry and Shaw were members of the Government's Advisory Committee on Pesticides. Would they be able to act impartially? Their response was toxicologically naive and full of inaccuracies and misrepresentations of what I had said. For instance, they used data solely from the manufacturers of phosmet, instead of independent data. On the basis of this, they argued that phosmet would only contaminate the fat of treated animals and would not get into the liver, kidney and muscles, and thus would not get inside cells and would not make contact with prion protein and therefore not interact with it. Therefore, they argued that phosmet would be unlikely to play a role in the causation of BSE. However, I presented counter-evidence from peer-reviewed articles by several teams who had carried out experiments with phosmet. The articles demonstrated that phosmet, which is after all a systemic OP, does penetrate the liver, kidneys and muscles, at twice the intensity that it penetrates the fat. Yet the SEAC conclusions ignored this and took Professors Shaw's and Berry's evidence from the manufacturers as gospel, and completely ignored my evidence.

I was also amazed that SEAC never considered the findings of the

Institute of Psychiatry, which was the prime motivating factor for the meeting.

The BSE Inquiry opened in March 1997 and I gave evidence on 26 March 1998. I was granted a full day to present my case. After the Inquiry had finished many commentators incorrectly summed up its conclusions on the link between OPs and BSE as being an outright dismissal. This was incorrect because Professor Malcolm Ferguson-Smith, the chief scientific advisor to the Inquiry, in his summing up that day called for more research into the subject, presumably because he thought the case had some merit. I basically agreed with the Inquiry's scientific summary that OPs were unlikely to be the sole cause of BSE. The Inquiry did however consider that it was plausible that OPs and other environmental factors might have played a role in the cause: '... a direct toxic effect of OPs on nerve cells seems an unlikely explanation for these diseases ... However, the finding that PrP (prions) can be modified in vitro by appropriate chemistry raises the possibility that similar reactions might be induced by environmental factors in vivo.' This latter sentence was crucial. It all hung on finding the 'appropriate chemistry'.

In early 2001 a committee headed by Professor Gabriel Horne was commissioned by the Government to reinvestigate the origins of BSE and they published their findings in the late summer of that year. In my view this involved the Government publishing incorrect information. After receiving the committee's report I approached DEFRA over the misrepresentations and errors and informed them that if they didn't amend their document I would sue them.

The report was defamatory in relation to the credibility of my work. It prejudiced my professional integrity and reputation as an international TSE researcher and lecturer, as well as my capacity to generate grant funding for research projects and to provide an income.

I received a letter from their legal department, dated 1 November 2001, which informed me that they were considering my comments and hoped to be in a position to respond shortly. I heard nothing after that date, nor have any of the amendments that I requested been applied to the DEFRA publication in question.

The Horne Report: scrutinizing the scrutineers

The Horne publication sought to separate the key OP and mineral facets of my multifactorial theory and then to treat each as entirely separate theories. It's an age-old trick — misquote the theory at the start in order to demolish it (no one but the author will notice!).

The approach of this committee followed a politically manipulative rather than scientifically based methodology. The report betrays its unilateral, prejudiced perspective by employing unscientific methodology to support the Establishment's theory, by repeated use of personal communications and unpublished papers as text references; any personal communications or unpublished papers that were presented as evidence in support of the dissident theories were entirely discounted.

It is clear that this committee had no genuine intention to uncover the true origins of BSE, but were more concerned about cementing a firmer foothold on the conventional Establishment theory after the previous BSE Inquiry report (2000) had exposed so many flaws. There were seven main statements that I found unacceptable.

It has been suggested that OP pesticides may have been the primary cause of the BSE epidemic in the UK. OPs have been used worldwide for many years for control of ectoparasites in cattle.
I have never said that OPs for ectoparasites are involved in BSE. I blame systemic types of dithiophosphate OPs, which penetrate into the brain and spinal cord and are used exclusively at high concentrations in the UK for controlling endoparasites.

There is no direct experimental evidence to support or refute the proposed mechanisms of action.

The Inquiry team did consider the published findings of the experimental work carried out at the Institute of Psychiatry, which does support my theory. Their publication deliberately or through carelessness, omits to report half of the positive results of the study, which confirmed the increased period of retention of the prion protein on the cell membrane in the phosmet treated cells – a well-known hallmark of the prion diseased cell.

This required treatment of all infested animals with OPs (specifically phosmet which is described by Humphreys as a non-systemic insecticide). All warble fly insecticides had to be formulated as a 'systemic', oil-based liquid 'pour on' to enable them to penetrate both the skin of the cow and the cells of the fly larva in order to kill it. A non-systemic formulation of phosmet would fail to kill the warble fly due to lack of penetration.

Nearly all the cows that developed BSE were born after 1982 so were never treated with phosmet to eradicate warble fly.
Erroneous – 1982 was the year in which warble fly eradication first became compulsory, not the year in which it ceased. After 1982 MAFF were compelling phosmet treatment in the warble infested areas, as well as urging annual prophylactic treatment of all herds in the UK (whether residing in infested or non-infested areas) up until 1995.

Data supplied by the chemical industry to the first BSE Inquiry demonstrates that the toxic concentration of the phosmet brands on the market had gradually increased from 1972, when a 5% concentrated solution was first licensed, to December 1978, when a 20% concentrated solution was first approved. It is perhaps no surprise that BSE first broke out in the mid-1980s as a legacy of the first applications of the high concentration treatment in the early 1980s.

Guernsey, which had no official campaign against warble fly, had 669 cases of BSE. Jersey, which did officially treat cattle for warbles had only 138 cases.

Jersey never officially treated cattle for warbles – confirmed by the Jersey Government's chief vet officer, Noel Martin, in letters that he wrote to the farming press when NOAH (the veterinary insecticide industry's lobby group) first made this statement.

This committee didn't see the need to check the pesticide industry's incorrect claim. I had explained the differences between Guernsey and Jersey BSE as lying in the variation in the soil mineral content of the islands, manganese additives and voluntary use of phosmet for lice.

While some imbalances of trace element nutrition may have become more pronounced in recent years, none are unique to the UK.
This separates the trace element tenet of my theory from the organophosphate one. OP exposure will transform, by oxidation, CNS accumulations of manganese 2+ into the pro-oxidant manganese 3+ form, which triggers the free radical mediated chain reaction of neurodegeneration. Such an oxidative conversion will be greatly accelerated in animals that are already deficient in the antioxidants selenium, zinc and copper.

In addition the spatial distribution of areas of low copper and high manganese in topsoils do not coincide with the BSE incidence distribution in England.
My referenced argument was that the recent increase in manganese was partly through artificial supplementation of feeds, replacement calf milk powders and fertilizers and is not exclusively related to local soil levels of the mineral. DEFRA compared a map of the high manganese/low copper regions in the UK with three BSE maps, which only cover three years out of the total of 15 years of BSE. However, if you study the other 12 BSE maps, which cover the remaining 12 years, then you see a correlation between the total of 15 BSE maps and the high manganese/low copper UK soil map.

The Horne report was a poor piece of work, but somehow in spite of this it has become fixed as gospel, a matter of record. [Its legacy has followed Mark around, with his obituary writers, such as Steve Connor in the *Independent* and an anonymous author in the *Telegraph* using it to dismiss his work. – N.P.]

Three weeks before Labour came to power in 1997, the Labour spokesman on environmental protection, Michael Meacher, had written an article in the *Daily Telegraph* on 10 April 1997 entitled 'Let's find the real cause of BSE', in which he promises to tackle the use of insecticides on cattle. He wrote: 'A new government should sweep aside these evasions. The Purdey theory should now be taken very seriously by the authorities. It is high time that a full-scale research programme was instituted into the role that OPs may play, not only in BSE/CJD, but in the contribution they may make in the development of diseases such as ME, MS, Alzheimer's, Parkinson's, depression and heart disease.'

After Labour got in, however, it took six years of phone calls, brush-offs and letters until a meeting was finally fixed for Thursday, 15 May 2003. It wasn't Mr Meacher's fault, but it was his office, which drew out the arrangements. I finally met him, together with Lord Tom King, former Defence Minister, and told them about some of my striking new findings collected during my trip to the USA. They seemed keen to ensure that I was funded properly for my research, but then handed me over to the very same senior government officials in the chief science group who rejected my last grant application. There seemed to be an overriding misconception at the meeting that it was the peer-reviewers who had stymied my grant application, but I was quick to point out that it was the DEFRA officials who had rejected it, rather than the reviewers. Four of the five reviewers had actually come out in support of funding my three-year study, and DEFRA had run with the single negative review.

I was naive enough to have my fingers burnt again. My latest data was whisked away, publicly ridiculed and then ironically plagiarized by a 'tame' professor, appointed by DEFRA, and served up in a further application to the EU and given full funding.

I felt totally drained by this whole episode. Once again, it seems that the writers of the TV comedy *Yes, Minister* had it about right – the civil servants, as opposed to the ministers, have the real power.

BSE continued to blight UK farming well into the twenty-first century, albeit at decreasing levels. But there were still extra-ordinary outbreaks, such as on a remote Pembrokeshire farm. The *Farmer's Guardian* of 3 June 2005 reported that the UK's government experts are claiming that the remnants of contaminated feed in the holds of ships were to blame for the outbreaks of BSE on a Pembrokeshire farm in cows that were born as late as 2002. This is 14 years after the UK Government's 1988 total ban on meat and bone meal entering ruminant feed, and nine years after the second 'reinforced' ban. Boatloads of MBM, which contained the highest doses of infective material in the mid-to-late 80s, produced no cases of BSE in these importing countries. How can they claim that cross contamination from presumably homoeopathic doses of MBM residues left in the holds of these boats account for these most recent anomalous cases of BSE?

As considerably smaller outbreaks of BSE began to erupt across other European countries, and later Japan, my investigations revealed the voluntary usage of the same types of systemic insecti-cide in those countries, albeit at half the dose rates of the UK. The European outbreaks seemed to follow an EU campaign known as COST 811, which was aimed at purging the remaining bastions of warble infestation on the European mainland – countries where outbreaks had continued because their respective authorities had adopted a more laid back, voluntary approach towards the control of warbles.

The USA had wisely adopted a less toxic approach for dealing with their warbles. They employed lower doses of 'non-systemic' acting insecticides, which were not designed to penetrate the skin, whilst only treating the individual cattle which were warble infested. For example, the use of systemic phosmet at a 10 mg/kg of body weight dose is voluntarily practised for lice control in warble-free Australia and New Zealand. But BSE has probably never erupted in Australia because, unlike Europe, these countries don't incorporate manganese into their cattle feeds, nor do they over-fly livestock zones with supersonic turbojet military and passenger aircraft.

There have been five cases of BSE in Japan, which all occurred in herds raised along the coastal belt of northern Hokaiddo. This farming district has traditionally imported breeding stock from the warble-infested territories of North America. In order to maintain Japan's warble-free status in an area that is climatically well suited for warble flies, these herds are treated prophylactically with a 10 mg/kg dose of systemic OP trichlorphon warblecide. Furthermore, low-flying Japanese military jets patrol the coastal waters of north Hokaiddo, due to its closeness to Russian held territory.

The 10 mg/kg dose of systemic pour-on trichlorphon warblecide has been used for warble control in all the countries afflicted with a low incidence of endemic BSE such as Holland, Portugal, Switzerland, Japan, Italy, Germany, Spain and France. It was also used in the voluntary early stages of the UK and Eire's warble eradication campaigns.

Look after the coppers

An adequate supply of copper is essential for the prion protein to be correctly manufactured in a mammal's cells. This led me to theorize that the copper component of the protein plays a role in conducting electrical signals into the areas of the brain that are mediated by the 24-hour circadian (daylight–darkness) rhythm. Once the availability of copper falls below a certain level, then the protein will cease to fulfil its metabolic function of conduction.

An early inspiration for me was the work of Pattison and Kimberlin of MAFF. They had discovered that a copper chelating chemical called cuprizone created a spongiform encephalopathy in animals without the requirement of any infectious agent. This was an important precedent for showing how abnormal chemistry can produce this pathology. This type of encephalopathy turned out to be non-transmissible, but it begged the question that if there was a substitution by another metal microcrystal (through an environmental exposure) at the vacated copper sites on the prion protein the result might be a transmissible spongioform encephalopathy.

Besides the dithiophosphate OPs there are several other possible copper chelators in the farm environment, such as manganese dioxide feed additives, silver compounds and tributyltin contaminants, which should also be considered as possible candidates for diminishing copper within the CNS. Increased levels of molybdenum in the food chain of cattle could also bring about copper depletion by conjugating with copper. This could result from the increased incorporation of high molybdenum sorghum into concentrated cattle feeds or from grazing cattle on soil that has become progressively acidified due to the modern day effects of acid rain. Excessive irrigation or the overuse of some artificial nitrogen fertilizers renders molybdenum more freely 'available' for uptake into the plants.

The origins of the UK's BSE epidemic

Although OPs were probably not the sole cause of BSE, I was convinced that they played a major role in BSE causation. Since the 1930s OPs had been used as insecticides, although they were quite scarce in those days. The German military saw their 'potential' and developed them as neurotoxins for use in nerve gases. And they've been in common use since the 1960s, later usurping the organochlorine group of pesticides, such as DDT.

During the 1980s general exposure to pesticides would have increased the permeability of the blood-brain barriers of treated cows, thereby weakening the brain's defence against the uptake of toxic levels of metals.

The chemical structure of the warblecide dithiophosphate, phosmet, would act as a chelator of copper, the two free sulphur atoms of the dithiophosphate locking copper into a mercaptide ring, creating an artificially induced form of copper deficiency in the central nervous system. It would also compete for the sulphur bonding sites in some other key proteins, such as the sulphated proteoglycans.

The OP trichlorphon, which was used in many countries with low BSE incidence, doesn't chelate copper like phosmet, but it could disrupt copper bonding to the prion – a delayed toxic mechanism that has been specifically associated with trichlorphon-induced protein ageing.

Phosmet was basically doing, albeit more weakly, what cuprizone had done in Pattison's work. There was therefore still another factor necessary to make this pathology transmissible and this is where microcrystal contaminants came in. The simultaneous exposure of UK cattle to phosmet during the 1980s would have enabled any rogue metal microcrystals that contaminated the UK environment to enter the brain and then bind up with these proteins in place of their correct metal co-partner, initiating the TSE disease process.

Cluster buster

My results from worldwide research indicated that high levels of metal microcrystals, such as manganese, barium, strontium and silver, in combination with deficiencies of copper, zinc, natural sulphur and selenium constituted an abnormal mineral imbalance, which was common to every TSE cluster region that I analysed. The levels were normal in TSE-free adjoining areas. I also identified the presence of high intensities of low frequency sonic shockbursts in all of these TSE cluster environments, which stemmed from a variety of prominent sources, such as low flying military jets, Concorde, quarry and military/gun explosions, volcanic and earthquake tectonic rift lines, thunder and electric storms.

I found that wherever the key clusters of TSE have emerged there is a temporal connection to a significant source of metal contamination. The metals are emitted both from naturally occurring sources such as volcanic eruptions and by man-made activities such as quarrying and the extraction of rock, coal or oil, which are naturally rich in barium and strontium, from steel, glass, ceramic, welding, oil drilling, the military munitions industries, from personal exposures to dental amalgams and surgical instruments (the silver in depth electrodes), and from the use of barium in radiographic investigations or silver in water purification.

The seeds of mad-cow madness

The crystals leak across the blood-brain barrier, facilitated by the presence of other abnormal eco-influences, and penetrate into brain cells, which are low in copper and sulphur. They are then free to bond up with brain proteins, in place of their normal copper and sulphur co-partners, whereupon they seed the growth of large metal-protein crystal arrays. Once the microcrystals become lodged and bonded into the nerve membranes they start to multireplicate, growing into substantial metal-protein crystals, which form the characteristic fibrils of the TSE brain.

These crystals are 'piezoelectric' in nature and work much like the crystals used in vintage microphones. They convert the energy of incoming acoustic sound waves into electrical energy. If the brain becomes contaminated by these rogue crystals, it is no longer able to conduct and dissipate any high energy shockbursts of sound and light to which it is exposed.

The incoming energy absorbed by the crystals is subsequently converted into electrical shocks, which generate magnetic fields around the crystals and initiate chain reactions of free radical damage in the surrounding tissues. The additional impact of the radioactive decay emitted from the metal component of these crystals serves to compound the intensity of the chain reactions.

Spongiform neurodegeneration of the brain ensues, represented by the haloes or spongiform holes that surround these fibril structures in the TSE brain.

The piezoelectric crystal facet of this theory is supported by the classic hypersensitive response of the BSE affected cow to the vet's hand clap test, which is a useful field test for diagnosing clinical BSE in a suspect cow. If the cow has BSE, the modest shock waves of the hand clap will invariably cause the poor beast to collapse, quivering, bellowing and writhing in agony — as though the clap had detonated an electric shock inside the cow's brain.

My hypothesis is that the rogue metal microcrystal represents the transmissible, pathogenic agent that underpins TSEs. This explains many of the missing links in our understanding of these diseases, such as why TSE can be invoked by inoculation with inorganic ash from TSE brain material heated to 800°C. How can the various protein-only or microbiological agents that have been ascribed to the cause of TSEs begin to survive this temperature and retain their so-called hyperinfectious property?

The metal crystal nucleator can survive these high temperatures, and then be transmitted back into a healthy animal, where it can re-seed the pathogenic metal-protein crystals. The magnetic charge that is permanently captured within these ferrimagnetically ordered crystals will not be drained until temperatures are raised above the 'Curie point' of the specific metal involved — around 600°C for manganese. Furthermore, the structure of the crystals is retained until temperatures exceed their melting point, which can be as high as 1000°C for some crystal species. My thesis also explains how TSEs can sometimes be transmitted via blood transfusions or injections of pituitary growth hormone treatments where the rogue microcrystal contaminants are contained within the treatment material.

It is interesting that metals such as barium and strontium are actually exploited in therapeutics for 'seeding' the process of crystallization in bone matrix as a means of reversing the wasting of bone in osteoporosis. But under conditions of good health, the process of mineralization within the organism is under delicate bioregulation whereby any aberrant crystal growth is kept in check. But once this delicate regulatory system is disrupted, then diseases such as rheumatoid arthritis, Alzheimer's disease and TSEs are able to proliferate.

Concrete evidence

There was another major route through which microcrystals appeared in the farm food chain. Although never admitted in public, the UK Government haven't denied the reports by people living beside cement kilns that empty animal feed lorries were frequently pulling into these sites, loading up with the kiln dust and then departing to unknown destinations, presumably to animal feed mills. This was happening during the 1980s and early 1990s at a time when there was considerable research into the development and incorporation of the resulting kiln ash, known as aragonite, into all types of animal concentrated feeds. The aragonite was valued as an additive because it contained beneficial minerals such as calcium, although any animals that consumed it were unwittingly exposed to a cocktail of other metals such as strontium, barium and manganese, which were nutritionally less desirable. The feeding of aragonite provides another plausible route through which metal microcrystals could have entered the farm food chain and 'seeded' the UK epidemic of BSE.

Perhaps of greater relevance to the origins of BSE was the fact that during the same period the use of coal in cement kilns was gradually replaced by the use of a product known as 'cemfuel' – a cocktail of chemical wastes, which included solvents, pesticides, car tyres and unexploded munitions. So the toxic residues remaining in the kiln ash would contain heavy metals, which would contaminate any animal feed containing the dust as a raw material.

After the cold war, a substantial tonnage of chemical warfare acids, such as the piezoelectric picric acid crystals, needed to be disposed of after the warheads were decommissioned at ordnance factories, such as Puriton in Bridgewater. The unexploded ordnance and contaminated soil wastes were processed into sludge or 'secondary liquid fuels' and supposedly transported out by 50:50 government/private companies and then taken to cokeworks and cement kilns across the UK for controlled incineration. This practice was accelerated prior to the privatization of the UK ordnance factories in 1987.

The supportive data

I published in several peer-reviewed journals my own environmental analytical data on the elevation of manganese, barium, strontium and silver and deficiencies of copper in the TSE cluster ecosystems. Some follow-up laboratory studies, apart from the Institute of Psychiatry work, were conducted which also provided positive support for my hypothesis. For example, cell culture experiments performed at Cambridge University by Dr David Brown showed that the prion protein folded into its abnormal shaped, protease resistant conformation (the form that hallmarks the brains of those who have died of TSEs) after the cells were loaded with manganese and deprived of copper. Manganese was one of the metals which I had found to be at high level in some of the TSE cluster zones, together with low copper. The aberrant bonding of manganese onto the prion – in place of copper – was considered responsible for misfolding the protein into its abnormal form. This was published in the journal of the European Molecular Biology Organization.

Another study at the US prion disease surveillance centre at Case Western University, Ohio, demonstrated that CJD affected brain material contained a tenfold elevation in manganese and a 50% reduction in copper in relation to the brains of those who had died of non-neurological disorders.

Further work was conducted in Japan, at Kobe University, where exposure of manganese bonded prion protein to specific wavelengths of light had caused the metal proteins to aggregate into the aberrant fibril structures that hallmark the brains of TSE victims.

Some more interesting work which confirmed my position in respect of manganese/copper balance was published in 2005 by the South Korean scientist N.H. Kim. This was followed in 2006 by a paper in which Deloncle et al. of the Université François Rabelais de Tours showed that manganese could give a positive result in the Western blot prionics test.

The flaws in the official theory

In the early BSE years I met several farmers who had never used the incriminated feed on their farms and yet were getting cases of BSE, so I soon became deeply sceptical of the conventional views on the origins of BSE and its human equivalent, vCJD. As time went on, with the epidemiological perspective filling out, there was growing contra-evidence to both MAFF's and the Royal Society's theories.

The hyperinfectious hypothesis is based on a single strand of evidence, that TSEs can be transmitted, in a laboratory context, via injections of homogenized TSE diseased brain tissues into unfortunate experimental animals. In the real world, however, animals are not exposed in this way to TSE material. Science must be precise and to extrapolate from these experiments to deduce what occurs *in vivo* is a crucial mistake. This extrapolation was, to coin a popular phrase used by my detractors, 'junk science' because the lab trials don't replicate the dose, the preparation method or the exposure route encountered in the real world.

The key flaws in the hypotheses are exposed in the following evidence:

1. Hundreds of thousands of tons of the BSE incriminated meat and bone meal (MBM) feed were exported as cattle feed during the 1970s/1980s/1990s to countries whose cattle populations have remained BSE-free to date, e.g. South Africa, Sweden, Eastern Europe, the Middle East, India and the Third World. Why did this feed not cause BSE abroad?

2. Relaxation in the temperature and manufacturing techniques of the MBM rendering process in the UK was blamed for allowing the survival of the scrapie agent in the sheep brain material and thereby enabling the 'agent' to infect cattle, producing BSE. None of these alterations, however, were exclusive to the UK rendering plants, since other scrapie endemic countries such as the USA and Scandinavia had adopted the same 'continuous flow' system of rendering five years before the UK, yet these countries have remained BSE-free. Furthermore, the pathogenic, 'infectious' capacity of the scrapie agent has been shown to remain active after heating to temperatures up to 1000°C – way above the 150°C temperatures employed in the supposedly 'safe' rendering processes operating in pre-BSE days. Research that examined whether the acetone solvent extraction, which had been used before the relaxation, had inactivated the scrapie prion showed that it had virtually no effect on the prion's pathogenicity.

3. Forty thousand plus cows that were born after the UK's 1988 ban on MBM incorporation into cattle or other ruminant feed have still developed BSE.

4. These 40,000 misfit cases of BSE were partly blamed upon vertical transmission, e.g. transmission of the infectious prion from mother to calf. In an experiment at a Department of Agriculture farm at High Mowbray, BSE couldn't be induced in nearly 1000

calves/embryos, which were incubated and reared by mother cows maintained under high risk BSE conditions (according to the MBM theory). These 40,000 anomalous cases of BSE were partly blamed on vertical transmission of the infectious prion from mother to calf.

5. Several countries such as Ireland, Portugal and France have witnessed a greater number of BSE cases in cows born after their respective bans on MBM than in cows born before their bans.

6. There have been no cases of BSE in other TSE-susceptible ruminants in the UK, such as goats and sheep, despite the customary inclusion of the same BSE-incriminated MBM protein source in their feeds.

7. Four of the original five kudu antelope that developed BSE at the London Zoo had no possible access to MBM containing feeds.

8. The UK Government's former experimental farm at Liscombe on Exmoor was designed to raise suckler beef cattle on a pure grass/silage system – without resort to feeding any MBM containing concentrated feeds at all. Yet BSE struck down four animals on this holding.

9. It is customary for Icelandic sheep farmers to slaughter and eat their scrapie affected sheep (brains included) immediately the first symptoms of this rapid wasting disease are recognized. Yet no cases of CJD have ever been recorded in Icelandic sheep farmers, and there has been only two cases of CJD in the population of Iceland at large.

10. The infamous mechanically retrieved meat products and processed baby foods blamed for causing vCJD in the UK were exported all over the world to countries where vCJD has not erupted to date.

11. BSE caused by MBM ingestion fails to fulfil Koch's first postulate, that the disease organism must be observed in all cases of the disease: 10–30% of cattle that were slaughtered each month under the BSE slaughter order didn't exhibit 'infectious' prions (the supposed causal agent) in the post-mortem analyses of their brainstem samples. The identical symptoms and space/time distribution of

these so-called 'BSE negative' cases with the BSE positive cases suggests that the 'negative' cases were all part and parcel of the same disease.

It also fails to fulfil the third postulate, that a culture of the disease organism must be capable of reproducing the disease when inoculated into a suitable experimental animal. Several live animal trials in the USA failed to induce BSE in cattle after feeding or injecting them with massive doses of scrapie contaminated brain tissue. All known strains of scrapie were tried. Sheep remains have been added to cattle feed since the nineteenth century and cattle have cross-grazed pasture with sheep since scrapie was first recorded over 250 years ago, and therefore cattle have been exposed to scrapie for centuries.

A ten-year UK government trial failed to transmit BSE via the oral ingestion of MBM into 1000 experimental cows kept at their High Mowbray experimental farm. The irony was that thousands of cattle on the 'real' farms in the UK during this period, which weren't eating any MBM, were going down with BSE.

*

According to my research, the substantial drop off in the incidence of BSE during the late 1990s is due to a combination of environmental factors: the virtual eradication of the warble fly, with a corresponding cessation of use of the OP warble fly insecticides during the 1990s. Furthermore, cows which are more susceptible to these environmental challenges were more susceptible to BSE and have died as a result before they calved, leaving the less susceptible animals alive.

Twenty-two years on and BSE still occurs in the UK, with around a hundred confirmed cases occurring in 2006.

2

The Crystal Grail

The prospect of the emergence of BSE in humans had hung over the British nation for many years since BSE had first erupted in the UK in the mid-1980s. In May 1995 it became a reality; a disease that had affected hundreds of thousands of UK cattle had claimed its first human victim, 19-year-old Stephen Churchill. The disease was a new variant of the very rare sporadic Creutzfeldt-Jakob disease (CJD) and was to become known as variant (v)CJD.

CJD is the most common of the human TSEs and exists in three forms: the sporadic, which has an unknown cause and occurs at the rate of about one case per million every 1–2 years; familial cases, which are associated with a mutation in the prion gene; and iatrogenic cases, which result from accidental transmission via contaminated surgical equipment or as a result of cornea or dura mater transplants or the administration of human-derived pituitary growth hormones. In contrast to the other forms of CJD, vCJD has affected much younger people and the disease progression is much quicker.

On occasions when there are more 'unknowns' than 'knowns' surrounding the official explanation for the cause of a novel disease such as vCJD, the climate becomes ripe for paranoid and hysterical speculation. It was not surprising that the statements of microbiologists such as Professor Richard Lacey and Dr Stephen Dealler were projected across the front pages of the national newspapers on an almost daily basis. Predictions of 'human BSE' (vCJD) were commonly referred to as an up and coming 'disaster of biblical proportions'.

Given the horrific images of BSE suffering cows that had been so frequently shown on our TV screens, it was understandable that the public were going to ask questions and demand that their health authorities take a note of all perspectives of the emerging science on BSE. But in light of the uncertainties that continued to surround the causes, controls and treatments for this disease, the momentum of the hyperinfectious myth was rapidly building.

Whilst my own personal research and observations on the farm didn't square with the science of Lacey and others – for a multitude of reasons – no one could deny that the 'infectious' hypothesis had raised important perspectives that needed to be addressed. It was clear the theoretical transmissible facet of these diseases could not be ignored, particularly when potentially millions of humans were consuming beef products that contained some abnormal prion material. Would these food products transmit the disease when eaten? No one knew for sure. I did agree with the authorities that the precautionary principle should prevail and that the intro-duction of some of the bans was the correct thing to do at the time. The first ban was introduced in November 1989 on the use of specified bovine offal in human food. The second ban followed in November 1995 on mechanically recovered meat, used in pies and hamburgers. From April 1996 the sale for human consumption of meat from cattle aged over 30 months at the time of slaughter was prohibited. Finally, in December 1997, the 'beef-on-the-bone' ban was introduced.

One thing was clear, the UK Government had become saturated by the vested interests of the meat and livestock industry. They were wilfully disregarding the science of any detractor who posed a threat to the official line on BSE and vCJD. It was not surprising whistle-blowers, such as Professor Lacey, were given the same short shrift which I had been subjected to.

Such a dismissive approach by the Government was entirely wrong; they should have been pulling out all the stops to get to the root of the disease, and basing their preliminary investigations on a full perspective of research. They should also have been aware of the gaps in their knowledge, and recognized the importance of plausible bursts of insight that were flowing from the farmers and vets who were, through their direct experience, familiar with the full case histories of BSE suffering cattle.

When the first case of vCJD occurred in 19-year-old Stephen Churchill from Devizes in Wiltshire everyone was truly shocked. The realities of this new disease and the merciless manner in which the symptoms of degeneration quickly conquered its victims were unprecedented. The sight of trembling cows in the advanced stages of neurological disintegration on the TV screen was one thing, but the harsh realities of such a grotesque condition affecting teenagers, possibly on a grand scale, posed an almost unbearable prospect for the nation.

My early surveillance of the environments of the vCJD clusters soon unearthed some common denominators and I soon parted company with the ideas of Richard Lacey and others. In fact, I increasingly found contra-evidence to their theories. They failed to substantiate their view that vCJD victims had contracted the disease as a result of consuming BSE contaminated beef. Because of the very common rural clustering of the cases it made more sense to me that vCJD had emerged in individuals who had been exposed to the same rare combination of environmental factors that had caused BSE. Where vCJD was concerned I was becoming interested in the possible role of the metal silicate microcrystals in the disease. Would I find the presence of glass, munition, steel, cement, brick and tile related industries at the centres of the CJD clusters and some especially potent species of silicate that could account for the aggressive nature of the vCJD?

What was so unusual about the emergence of vCJD was that it was occurring in low population density village communities, often in the same road, with victims sometimes even knowing each other and even sharing homes (the incidence has thankfully been very, very low). We were soon told that eating infected beef products was the likely cause of vCJD. In effect this would mean that most of the 60 million people in the UK, together with several million visitors and consumers of exported beef products (exported products, being processed, are likely to contain higher doses of the incriminated prion material) would have had at least some exposure. There is still no published trial in which food products, such as burgers, containing incriminated beef have produced a TSE or anything like it in an experimental animal.

The majority of the 170 cases of vCJD recorded to date have involved people who were raised or spent time in the rural and coastal communities of the UK. Since beef is consumed equally between town and country people alike, the beef hypothesis is not supported by the predominantly rural upbringing of the vCJD victims. Several CJD epidemiologists have made reference to data that demonstrate a larger proportion of CJD victims have pursued professions or hobbies that are practised outdoors in rural environments, e.g. farming, forestry, kennel work, horticulture, stable work, coastguards, the military, horse riding, fishing, exercising pets, shooting, cross country running and outdoor sports.

The CJD Surveillance Unit at Edinburgh has identified nine geographical locations in the UK where two or more spatially associated cases of vCJD had co-emerged but their investigations could not identify any common causal association between these regions and their relationship to beef consumption. For example, a 1975 study by W.B. Matthews on the distribution of sporadic CJD cases in England and Wales from 1964 to 1973 reported that nearly half of the total CJD incidences in the UK involved people who were living in rural areas at the time of onset of the disease. He also reported: 'Several geographical clusters of CJD were identified, none of them related to areas of dense urban population'. He also noted that it was 'remarkable that three cases of this rare disease have occurred in a small community'; any modern day repeat of this occurrence is casually outcast as a coincidence and thus not fully researched by the health authorities for as long as they can get away with it. Furthermore, use of the term 'cluster' is conveniently avoided until five or more cases have occurred in a small community.

Another important, though bizarre epidemiological factor surrounding these mini-clusters of vCJD involved a number of
instances when more than one case of vCJD had broken out in the
same street of the small community involved. It was almost as
though we were really confronting a very selective infection, caused
by a highly contagious agent. And yet this was not convincing
because if the disease was infectious why did it never spread to
family members? It was much more plausible that we were looking
at a select group of environmental factors whose co-occurrence was
very rare. Despite the confidentiality over the location of the 'same
street' outbreaks, the media had ascertained that the villages of
Armthorpe, Queniborough, Eastleigh, Adswood and Lympstone
were all involved. In the case of Queniborough, what was even more
interesting was that in one road in which two vCJD cases occurred
there had been one case of sporadic CJD approximately ten years
earlier.

In some of the other mini-clusters, the individual victims were
known to have gone to the same school, shared a childhood
friendship or shared the same flat. The same degree of inter-
relationship between victims has also been demonstrated in the
clusters of conventional sporadic CJD, but the need to identify an
explanation for this mysterious phenomenon has long been put to
bed.

But the UK health authorities will not be drawn into a debate over
these bizarre occurrences. They have chosen to put them down to a
series of coincidences – an acceptable deviation from the norm,
which their 'all important' statistical modelling will allow for from
time to time. But when you are dealing with such an extremely rare
disease that is running at 1–2 cases per million head of population
per year, their dismissive approach to this 'golden opportunity for
useful investigation' is both irresponsible and nonsensical from a
public health and epidemiological perspective. In fact once the
public health issue of CJD became so highly politicized after the first
cases of vCJD broke out in the mid-1990s the criteria for deter-

mining what defines a 'cluster', i.e. the number of cases per square metre of residential area, seemed to mysteriously expand overnight.

One of the most moving testimonies at the public hearings of the BSE Inquiry was made by Roger Tomkins, in which he described the suffering with variant CJD of his daughter Clare, who died aged 24. In one sense it was good that the BSE Inquiry was launched on such a hard-hitting note. It had made the world fully aware of the anguish and despair that this young woman and her family endured, and of the cruel and relentless momentum of this new fatal disease. I remember my own reactions of horror towards the first symptoms of BSE in my cows, and I therefore had great admiration for Mr Tomkins, who, coping with infinitely greater horrors than my own, had the courage to deliver such a sensitive testimony in such a high profile public forum.

He had stood up in front of a full house and bravely described the course of neurodegeneration of his 'darling daughter', a one-time 'stunning, strawberry blonde with a personality to match'. Clare, who had been a vegetarian since 1985 from the age of 13, had been displaying some peculiar symptoms since early 1996, notably complaining of an odd taste in her mouth. When she returned from a holiday in October with her fiancé she was uncharacteristically depressed. She began to lose weight, became more depressed, to the point where she was crying for no reason, and she could no longer face her job in the pet department of a local garden centre. After only a few weeks of suffering from vCJD she deteriorated into a decrepit state, became bedridden, clinically blind and in constant danger of drowning in her saliva. Her family doctor and specialists had all thought that the cause of her condition was mental rather than physical. This was strange, given that one year previously the Government had written to psychiatrists asking them to look out for a particular group of symptoms that were associated with vCJD. Despite this, the psychiatrist treating Clare insisted that her symptoms of weight loss, crying, numbness, agitation and erratic behaviour were caused by a psychiatric illness. She was prescribed 'reward therapy', which provided her with treats, such as watching television whenever she made an attempt to look after herself and regain her self-esteem. Her family was not allowed to visit her during this dark period of therapy. Mr Tomkins told the Inquiry that he couldn't conceive of any reward that would motivate his daughter during her present condition. Not long after the start of the therapy, the family was told that her condition had worsened and they went to the hospital to find her in a totally exhausted state. 'Her skin was covered in carpet burns and her whole body in tiny cuts from the bed springs. Her terror and anxiety had caused her to self-inflict these injuries. She would hide under her bed. As her illness worsened, her hands turned inwards, her feet too. She became knock kneed and her hips disjointed, so she could not walk. Sometimes at night, she would howl like a sick, injured animal. She started to hallucinate. It was now clear to me that she was tormented in her condition.'

Not long after the BSE Inquiry concluded, I was contacted by Mr and Mrs Griffin, the parents of a recent vCJD victim, Leon, who lived not far from me at Burnham-on-Sea. As I started to interview Sandra, Leon's mother, a photo of Leon on the mantelpiece glinted in the morning sun and made a strong presence in the room.

Like most of the other vCJD families, Sandra was very frustrated by the way that the health authorities had treated her. Many parents had felt that their children were used as guinea pigs and singled out as hot property by medics who subjected them to a series of tests, which appeared to be more to do with advancing their academic careers than actually developing effective treatments. At the other extreme, the non-specialist health workers would regard vCJD patients as 'lepers', often refusing to get involved with them at any level. They feared infection with a 'lethal contagion', akin to AIDS, which was perhaps understandable considering the misinformation which the media had put out on vCJD. Victims were literally sent home to die from what was officially deemed to be an incurable or untreatable condition, which was outrageous considering the well-known beneficial effects which the sulphated proteoglycan molecules, such as pentosan polysulphate, had invoked in trials on TSE affected mice. The Simms family from Belfast saw the potential of this treatment and campaigned on behalf of their son, who had vCJD. In the end they had to sue the NHS and eventually won permission in London's High Court to proceed with the experimental pentosan polysulphate, available in the USA for the treatment of interstitial cystitis. The treatment eventually took place at a Belfast hospital and proved effective at slowing the disease down.

Sandra's answers to my questions about Leon threw up some interesting points, which reinforced the possible relevance of some of my findings from the cluster areas abroad. Much like Clare Tomkins, Leon had virtually lived a vegetarian lifestyle, choosing to eat plenty of apples and fresh vegetables. I then began to realize why the Griffins had been taking an interest in my position on the cause of TSEs. Leon had been studying in Salisbury at a college that is located in a major militarized area with a plethora of practice ranges on the Salisbury plain. It was during Leon's short stay at Salisbury that the first symptoms of vCJD had become apparent to his parents. Leon had driven off in the wrong direction after leaving college to return home. This squared with my observations of BSE suffering cows on my farm, which had suddenly forgotten the route of return to the milking parlour – a route which they had travelled over 700 times per year.

When Sandra disappeared for a moment to make a pot of tea, I stared out across the great flat expanse of the Somerset Levels, and watched the wind parting the canopies of some distant willow trees. For a moment I thought I could just pick out the chimney of the massive World War II ordnance factory, which was sited some four miles across the meadows at Puriton.

When Sandra came back, she described how Leon's eyes had changed colour to a grey-green during the early stages of the disease, one of the classic symptoms that could result from various types of metal intoxication. She also told me about Leon's habit of drinking Earl Grey tea, which contains a well-known photo-sensitizing agent called bergamot. It increases a person's sensitivity to the oxidative effects of ultraviolet light, which was a phenomenon I had identified as a common factor in many of my cluster studies. In fact, one of the Italian villages that had been blighted by 20 cases of sporadic CJD was actually located in the middle of a bergamot orchard. Likewise, the British dairy herd had been fed large amounts of citrus fruit pulp during the BSE era, the rind of which contains the furocoumarin that is responsible for the photo-sensitizing effect of citrus. I became intrigued by these seemingly insignificant threads of information, which might perhaps provide more clues to the riddle of TSEs.

The vCJD clusters

In the summer of 1999 I made my first trip into the cluster terri-tories of vCJD in the UK and it was to create a new dimension in my research. My brother and I started with the largest cluster, which had occurred in a charming village called Queniborough, a few miles north-east of Leicester. Our car turned the corner into a crooked lane that ran through endless stubble fields. I focused determinedly on the distant spire of Queniborough church, which dominated the open horizon, serving as an ideal orientation point for newcomers travelling to the village. As we turned into the high street, I was wondering what environmental features were unique to the village in relation to its neighbours. The official verdict on the death of five young people from vCJD who were connected to Queniborough was drawn up by Drs Monk and Bryant of the Leicestershire Health Authority. They stated that the traditional practice of skull splitting during the butchery process at the local butcher's shop had lead to the contamination (surely they meant additional contamination) of meat with central nerve tissues sourced from BSE affected carcasses. Firstly, skull splitting was not unique to the village butcher. It had been carried out at hundreds of traditional butchers throughout the UK. Secondly the quantity of additional infective material likely to pass into the human food chain would be infinitesimal. Why had no other clusters of vCJD cases erupted in all of the other villages whose local butchers applied the skull splitting practice? This theory was a non-starter and had failed to identify any plausible causal factors for the outbreak of vCJD in the village.

I went to speak to Mr Bramley, the butcher, whose traditional shop took the centre stage in the middle of the picturesque village high street. It was clear from the outset that he was well accustomed to being harassed by the media and other CJD investigators, so he was not surprisingly reluctant to engage with an outsider like myself in a discussion about vCJD. When I raised the subject, he became instantly anxious and on the defensive, although he relaxed considerably once he got the gist of my approach.

As we chatted, he recounted some of his experiences of persecution, where, for example, cars had driven past in the middle of the night with people screaming out 'murderer'. He even told me that the official inquiry officers had never even interviewed him. It seemed unfair that such a dedicated family businessman, with obvious high standards, had become a scapegoat in this complex medico-political affair as a result of the academic ignorance that surrounded BSE.

We went on to meet Rosemary and Bob Smith, a local couple who had a wide knowledge of local history. They guided us around the immediate environments of the vCJD homes in order that we could collect samples of the soil, vegetation and drinking water. After discussions with several other villagers, I focused on some sources of potential metal pollution in the parish. I also discovered that vCJD was not the only brain disease that was at high incidence in the area. One shopkeeper told me that there were apparently 11 cases of CFS/ME in those who lived in the houses that lay on the southern side of the village high street.

My first line of investigation centred on a former dye works, which, according to local people, had subjected the village, and the paint work of their cars in particular, to a regular showering of a yellow dust during the 1980s. A major fire broke out at the plant, worsening the contamination and shortly afterwards it closed.

Exposure to dyes had featured as one of the main TSE risk factors during my global survey, and there was a possibility that this short term exposure to either strontium yellow or picric acid (the piezo-electric yellow dye material that is also used as a detonator) was a causal factor.

There were other reports of a yellow dust with a sulphurous smell, which had regularly been deposited over the Queniborough district prior to the mid-1980s. This had been ascribed to the substantial operations of the iron industry operating to the north, around Corby, and the pollution from this plant must have implicated a much wider area than the vCJD cluster zone.

Another possible toxic metal source was the copious use of manganese-based fertilizers and fungicide sprays by the local arable farmers in the Queniborough area. The porous sandy soils in the district indicate that manganese and other trace elements are continually leached out by rainfall, and end up being present only at very low levels in the soil. In order to grow productive yields of arable crops, the farmers need to address this deficit by applying liquid manganese fertilizer and fungicide sprays throughout the growing season.

The recent trend in this type of agri-technology has been to design spray formulations where micro-particles of the active ingredient, such as manganese, are employed to guarantee an efficient penetration of the metal into the plant tissues. Unfortunately, use of these nanotech sprays will also guarantee a more efficient uptake of the metal into the tissues of any person who gets exposed to the atmospheric spray drift during the spray operations. However, although exposure of the local populations to these manganese sprays has undoubtedly increased over recent years, one would have expected a consistent increase in the number of vCJD cases emerging as a direct result. But the opposite has been the case.

I was exasperated when I eventually read the only counter-argument that the local Health Authority had mustered to answer my theory of metal-induced vCJD in Queniborough. In contrast to my own analytical test results, they had solely relied on the soil maps produced by the British Geological Survey to determine the levels of manganese in the village environment. How soil maps could possibly indicate the presence of an extremely localized source of metal pollution, which had probably developed after the publication of the map, was beyond my comprehension. They were obviously unaware of the need to use manganese sprays, which generate high levels of airborne manganese, to address the deficiency. The response was predictable: 'since manganese is not in the soil, then where does Purdey think the damn manganese is coming from – their Wellington boots!' That was the last I heard from the Leicestershire Health Authority.

Another exclusive pollutant feature that has dominated this part of the Leicestershire landscape for many years involves the emissions from the chimneys of a gypsum factory that has been manufacturing several types of plasterboard, which utilize barium and silicate based raw materials. Gypsum had also featured as a risk factor in the TSE cluster areas of Colorado and Sicily/Sardinia.

Perhaps the most intensive, relevant source of silicaceous microcrystal contamination in the vicinity stemmed from the World War II Queniborough ordnance depot, a 140 acre site to the northwest of the village, where East Goscote stands today.

Queniborough has the largest cluster of vCJD in the world, since five cases of this disease have been connected to this region. Once again, many of the victims had either lived in or been connected to a single street, known as the Ringway, a horseshoe-shaped avenue of post-war semi-detached homes. One of the victims lived in the road, another visited a relative who lived in the road, but there was also a case of sporadic CJD in the road occurring approximately ten years earlier. It surely cannot be a coincidence that these related diseases occur in the same road. Surely this scenario points to the victims being exposed to the same contaminants that were extant well before the sporadic CJD case, but with an additional factor promoting the variant form of the illness.

All of the Queniborough victims had grown up or played around the village and consumed wild game/fish/fruit grown around the site of the former ordnance depot, which had processed and stored chemical weapons right up until the 1960s. These would have included persistent types of chemical such as phosgene, mustard gas and other 'undisclosed' types of munitions, triggers and detonators. During World War II, these munitions had actually been stored along the verges of the lanes around Queniborough where the victims had regularly walked and rode their horses, in an attempt to avoid the possibility of being hit by the German bombing sorties.

The local community had free access to the site to hunt rabbits and pheasants and to eat the wild fruit that had grown on the site over the years. They had also caught fish, which had been raised in the lakes and Queniborough brook, which were fed by the drainage from the former ordnance site. People who worked at the top secret ordnance factory had also reported explosions, and on one occasion it was actually attacked by German bombers. When the depot came to be demolished in the 1960s, the works must have exacerbated the whole problem of microcrystal pollution by churning up dust clouds of microcrystals into the atmosphere.

The truth about the site was revealed when I came across a declassified copy of a map and photo of the depot, which had been published in a book about wartime Leicestershire. I was also able to see some photos of this site in the local council offices and these illustrated the substantial and intricate nature of the complex of buildings at the depot. This made it hard to believe that the site had never been used. But back in the 1960s nobody had asked questions about its true history, and the village of East Goscote was subsequently built over it. I later met some of the villagers, including some of the surviving Italian workers, who had been employed in the actual manufacture of the munitions at the depot. I remained amazed that the Government had so successfully maintained a cloak of secrecy surrounding the activities of the site right up until the present day.

But one or two of the pensioners seemed aware of its development into a military depot during the early1940s. These odd bursts of recollection from the local people had whetted my appetite for further investigation, although the majority of local intelligence was adamant that 'the depot had never been used for the purpose that it was intended, namely, a munitions depot'.

In the 1960s planning permission was sought to develop the redundant site as a new village, which would become known as East Goscote.

In 1962 Edward Anderson, an engineer for Barrow and Soar District Council, made a planning appeal to the Minister of Housing to grant permission for a new village to be constructed on land where a Royal Army ordnance depot had been built at the end of World War II. During the appeal the land was described as 'an obnoxious and loathsome eyesore to the landscape, the site being open to the Melton road, and having no barrier such as a hedge in order to obscure its ugliness from view'. If the local people had known the story of this seemingly innocuous piece of waste ground, their derogatory comments would have probably gone a lot further.

Nonetheless, planning permission was granted and a housing development company moved in and demolished what turned out to be a massive infrastructure of concrete bunker buildings, which covered the entire 140 acres. One monstrous building, which turned out to be the shell filling factory, had reinforced concrete blast walls four feet thick and these had proved impossible to demolish with the 'forever faithful' ball and chain concrete buster. Consequently, they were forced to bulldoze all of the rubble from the other buildings and literally bury the entire factory in a heap of rubble.

All that remains of the factory today are the two mounds that stand in the middle of East Goscote. During this demolition and again during excavations for the new village there would have been considerable exacerbation of silicaceous dusts. The rubble from the ordnance site may well have been used as a convenient and cheap source of hardcore in the development of East Goscote and at the Ringway in Queniborough. It is interesting that the Ringway road built at about this time lies only 1 km south-east across the fields of East Goscote, with Queniborough brook at its head. Another set of incidents involved the crash landings of two USAF Lincoln bomber aircraft in Queniborough during World War II. Both of the planes were overloaded with bombs and had exploded on impact, leaving gigantic craters in a couple of local farms in an area in which two victims, Chris Reeves and Pamela Beyless, had worked and had been horse riding respectively. When I spoke to one of the parents of a vCJD victim, they told me that they had first dated each other in 'the tunnels', i.e. the chambers of the former shell filling factory before they were properly filled in. They were totally uninformed about the former use of this underground chamber, and even today the children's slide in the playground at East Goscote is sited directly across the former entranceway into the chambers where the chemical weapons were assembled.

In 1961 the local council purchased two of the concrete reservoirs, which had been used in the production of chemical weapons, for the purpose of sewage sludge treatment. The development became known as the Wanlip sewage farm, which trucked out a continuous supply of sewage fertilizer for treating all of the farms that lay within a two to three mile radius of the site. The upshot was that all the farms within the parish of Queniborough were sprayed with the sludge on an almost annual basis, until the levels of toxic metals in the soil became so high that sewage spreading had to be restricted in 1985. It seems that a toxic cocktail of heavy metals was present in this sewage material from both the munitions residues and from the excessive amount of silicate textile waste that was discharged into the sewage system in this part of Leicestershire.

Perhaps it is no surprise that three victims of vCJD, Glen Day, Stacy Robinson and Chris Reeves, had used a particular footpath that crossed the sewage-treated fields to get to the Wreake Valley school. Furthermore, villagers had informed us how their homes were enveloped in a fine mist of sewage vapour every time the sewage operations were in full swing. I personally experienced this obnoxious phenomenon during one of my visits to the village! One of the vCJD families had regularly purchased a special 'garden fertilizer' brand of dried sewage sludge from the Wanlip works. They had incorporated this material into their garden soil to grow their vegetables. Once again, the Queniborough environment demonstrated its potential for contaminating its local population with microcrystals.

When I asked Rosemary and Bob Smith about the levels of acoustic shock around the village, they gave me the answer that seemed to explain why and when Queniborough suffered its outbreak of vCJD.

The secondary 'acoustic shock' prerequisite of my theory is also evident in Queniborough, because the Royal Air Force used the church spire as a marker for low flying jet training throughout the 1980s. The shock waves from the overflights could have activated the latent piezoelectric potential of any metal-protein crystals carried in the brains of contaminated individuals. This may help explain why vicars as an occupational group are blighted by the highest incidence of sporadic CJD (7 cases per million). Other factors that are relevant to this statistic are that vicars may also have more potential exposure to metal ions in the silver of the communion chalice, contamination from old metal organ pipes, the sound from the church bells and organ amplified in the 'resonating chamber' of the church. Yet another source of microcrystals and acoustic shock lies 6km to the west, in the village of Mountsorrel, where the largest granite quarry in Europe is sited. Local villagers report hearing the explosions which blast the granite from the quarry face.

Interestingly, Winston Churchill had ordered the mass manufacture and stockpiling of considerable tonnages of chemical weapons that were to be used as a last resort to defeat the Germans if the need had arisen. Fortunately, they were never used. These weapons were manufactured at Queniborough, Randle and Rock Savage in Cheshire and Springfields in Lancashire and dispersed to munitions stores (usually sited in woodland) close to airbases all along the east coast of the UK from Lossiemouth to Kent, as well as in North Wales.

After World War II, canisters containing approximately 17,000 tons of the organophosphate nerve gases sarin and tabun, 14,000 tons of phosgene, 120,000 tons of mustard gas, as well as other waste munitions (white phosphorus, etc.) and propellants (nitroglycerine) were removed from Queniborough and other ordnance and storage depots. They were then shipped out and dumped along fault lines such as the Beaufort Dyke, under the Irish and North Seas — areas which have been intensively trawled for the provision of fish protein for both human and livestock consumption in the UK.

The gradual corrosion of these canisters by sea water or mechanical damage, due to the laying of cables on the sea bed, has lead to reports of munitions leaking into the open seas over recent years. Fishermen have suffered acute intoxication as a result — indicating the start of a wide-scale contamination of the local marine food chain. Furthermore, corroding canisters containing white phosphorous and mustard gas munitions have been washed up on Irish and UK beaches since the late 1980s. Phosphorus represents one of the nucleating agents that can seed metal-protein crystals in biological tissues.

But UK government analyses of sea bed sediment and the 'edible' portion of fish has been unable to identify the parent compounds of the particular types of chemical munitions that were dumped in these seas. It should however be noted that this study failed to analyse the samples for the specific metabolites that are known to degrade via alkaline hydrolysis from these types of chemical ordnance. Thousands of tons of the 'inedible' fraction of fish – the bones and various organs, which would have bio-concentrated any metal pollutants – were directed into UK livestock feeds as a source of protein during the BSE era, particularly after meat and bone meal was ironically banned in 1988. But the use of fishmeal as a feeding-stuff has been considerably restricted since the mid-1990s for conservation reasons, and this drop in usage correlates with the considerable drop in rates of BSE incidence during this period.

The intensive feeding of fishmeal protein to the Icelandic sheep population during the winter months could also offer a plausible contributory factor as to why Iceland has the highest global incidence of scrapie. The same use of fishmeal feed applies to the Mediterranean sheep flocks affected with scrapie. Long term dumping of both chemical and conventional munitions and military radioactive waste on the sea bed around the coasts of Iceland and southern Italy is well recognized. Likewise, other animal species fed substantial amounts of fishmeal derived from the North Atlantic seas, such as mink, have also endured outbreaks of TSEs.

In respect of CJD incidence, fish, as opposed to beef, represents a more convincing candidate in the multifactorial aetiology of BSE and vCJD. It is also interesting that all cows that were home reared on fully converted organic farms have remained totally BSE-free, and organic farming standards had debarred the use of fishmeal as feed during the 1980s.

Whilst I was lecturing in Derby my brother went on to the former pit village of Armthorpe, near Doncaster, where there have been three cases of vCJD: a 19-year-old trainee chef, Matthew Parker; Adrian Hodgkinson, a former RAF corporal; and Sarah Roberts, an accountant.

In common with several other sufferers Sarah Roberts's doctors first thought her condition was psychiatric and she was told to buck her ideas up or else she would end up in a psychiatric hospital. She rarely ate beef, preferring chicken. Both Matthew and Sarah belonged to a group of children that often played together on the fields opposite their homes. They lived only 100 yards apart in Wickett Hern Road, sited on the edge of the village adjacent to an area that had been undergoing extensive redevelopment of a light industrial nature.

For many years Adrian Hodgkinson, who lived elsewhere, regularly visited his grandmother's home on Sundays, which was situated only three streets away from Wickett Hern Road.

Most of the TSE risk factors are present in this area, such as a recent history of extensive development, with excavation for new roads and general construction. Nigel reported getting covered with silicaceous particles from the excavations, which got in his eyes and throat as he walked in the area of Wickett Hern Road. The historic map of the area revealed a possible munitions link in a mound near the road where excavation was going on, called 'Gunhills' (we haven't managed to trace any detail of what the name denotes).

The soil in the area is bunter/Triassic sandstone and greensand formations, which are all notoriously manganese deficient. However, the soils from two fields adjoining Wickett Hern Road showed excessive levels of manganese at 76 mg/l and 154 mg/l, and the vegetation from these fields again had excessive manganese levels of 577 mg/kg and 212.5 mg/kg. These exceedingly high levels of manganese recorded in low-manganese soil districts suggest that an industrial source such as a dye, brickworks or a fertilizer or an atmospheric source of manganese is causing high contamination of these areas. There is a former brick and tile works close by. A brickworks is also sited close to Adswood, on the outskirts of Manchester, where two vCJD victims lived only 250 metres apart.

Other vCJD hotspots in the UK have been identified. One such mini-cluster involved two victims who had lived in Lympstone, near Exmouth in Devon, a village that lies on the estuary of the River Exe.

Interestingly the map of the distribution of cases of sporadic CJD for the 1970–9 period also demonstrates a confluence of cases along this same estuarine stretch of the River Exe. Although the beef from the local Lympstone butcher had been officially blamed for the outbreaks, one of the victims was a Royal Marine who lived at the barracks in Lympstone. This theory seemed flawed from the start, since the Marine caterers had purchased their meat supplies from the big meat wholesalers, and not from the local butcher's shop. The quantity of meat required for one meal serving at the Marine camp would have used up the entire stocks of the local butcher's shop.

Once again, the cause of these two cases of vCJD in a small village community seemed to pivot on a shared exposure to environmental factors that were present within the Lympstone vicinity. This village was sited next to a top security Marine encampment whilst being little more than three miles distant from their practice ranges at Woodbury Common. My brother's analysis of the local geological bedrock, which was fully exposed along the estuary cliffs, recorded very high levels of 1946 ppm barium and 44322 ppm manganese in select pockets, indicating the elevation of these metal silicates in the local area. So the overall potential for microcrystal contamination in the environment around Lympstone was high.

Furthermore, when I first drove into the village, I noticed aeroplanes from nearby Exeter International Airport flying low over the village. This same flight path was used by the regular charter flights of Concorde for which enthusiasts were paying £1500 a time to be flown around the Bay of Biscay at supersonic speed. According to the local people, the low frequency screeching noise of Concorde's afterburner jets was deafening. Each time the plane flew along the route of the estuary, it rattled their doors and windows, scattering farm animals and scaring little children into a temporary state of frenzy. The noise of Concorde, along with the noise of the low flying military jets, which utilize the same afterburner propulsion technology, represents one of the most intensive artificial low frequency noises that pervades the modern environment.

In fact, taking charter flights on Concorde out of provincial air-ports was fast becoming a popular pastime. You could fly from many airports in the UK to exotic destinations throughout Europe and the world. A cutting from the *Sunday Express* illustrates that this was gaining popularity at the same time that the first cases of variant CJD were appearing in those populations which lived beneath the take-off and low-fly airspace of any planes which, like Concorde, were propelled by the afterburner jet.

Another cluster of vCJD worthy of mention involves three out-breaks in some remote villages scattered along the most intensively militarized coastline of the UK – the sandy strand of shoreline that skirts the south-western corner of Wales. All of the vCJD victims involved in this cluster had studied together at the same school in Tenby. One of the cases involved a young girl who was a trainee potter (intensive exposure to silicates in the potting/ceramic pro-fession). She had just moved into a flat in the village of Amroth, which was located on the most westerly extremity of the massive weapons testing range along Pendine Sands. The other cases lived in villages that abutted the north and western borders of the Pen-dine range. Once again the manufacture of munitions, as well as the testing, had been intensively practised along this corner of the Welsh coastline – perhaps more than anywhere else in the UK. In fact the whole stretch of coastline surrounding this cluster zone was Pembrey air weapons range, Pendine Sands, Penally shooting range, along with the extensive tank ranges at Manorbier and Castlemartin. At peak periods of practice, apparently the ground actually wobbles beneath your feet.

Much like the Bishopton ordnance factory up at Glasgow, the Pembrey ordnance factory was engaged in the production of sub-stantial tonnages of propellants and TNT. It was constructed on 500 acres of isolated sand dunes sited midway between Kidwelly and Llanelly. Ian Hay's story of the Pembrey factories states that 'its activities were kept in evidence night and day, first by reason of the yellowish nitrous fumes discharged from its tall chimneys, and secondly, by the occasional smoke and glare of burning TNT, extracted from the bombs and shells no longer fit for service'. Five cases of sporadic CJD emerged in the period between 1980 and 1984 a short distance away, in a north-westerly direction from the factory. It is feasible that contaminating microcrystalline dusts had blown over their homes and local people might also have consumed local meat, fruit and vegetables that had come from the 'fall-out' zone of the plant.

Essex CJD

The chemical munitions that remained at Queniborough after World War II were all transported for incineration or for direct dumping onto the sea beds of the North and Irish Seas, as well as the coastal areas of Bawdsey and Aldburgh in Suffolk and Shoeburyness on the Essex coast. There was a massive munitions incinerator at Shoeburyness, as well as a substantial military firing range that is still in use today.

Interestingly, the area west of Shoeburyness has shown CJD clustering for many years. One of these clusters involved a well-documented outbreak of five cases within the Chelmsford, Billericay, Basildon, Southend districts during the 1970–9 period, with a further six cases during the 1980–4 period who had lived more directly around the Shoeburyness peninsular. More recently, the CJD surveillance group in Edinburgh reported 18 cases of CJD in Essex, between 1990 and 2001.

Likewise, during the period 1970–9 there was another cluster of four cases of CJD a few miles inland from the Bawdsey/Aldeburgh region – the other area where the Queniborough munitions were taken.

Sarah Ridgewell contacted me after seeing my BBC 2 film *Mad Cows and an Englishman*. Her family had lived at Maldon where Sarah's father had spent much of his leisure time sailing with his children in the Blackwater estuary; the river directly abuts the Shoeburyness peninsula. Sarah's father had developed a mutation on the prion gene, and was the first of her family to die of CJD. Two of Sarah's sibling's have subsequently died of familial CJD and now Sarah herself is purportedly suffering from the early stages of the disease.

When I interviewed her about her father's life, she immediately mentioned the key risk factors that I had found. Her father had served on the Royal Air Force bombers in the Far East during World War II, and had later brought his family to live in the Shoeburyness region. Sarah recounted how the foundations of her childhood home in Maldon were continually vibrating whenever the low frequency thump of the guns at Shoeburyness were in action. A combination of the fall-out of metal microcrystals (depleted uranium, barium, silver) and exposure to the sonic shocks from the range has in my opinion rendered the local communities at an increased risk of developing CJD.

Much like the other major TSE cluster areas in Slovakia, Calabria and Japan, the Shoeburyness area has produced all types of TSE which are co-emerging in the same areas, presumably indicating that all forms of TSE are essentially caused by the shared exposure to the same multifactorial environmental factors.

There have been about 170 cases of vCJD in Britain. The incidence is much lower abroad with 15 cases in France, four in Ireland, two in the US, and one each in Canada, Italy, Japan, the Netherlands, Portugal, Saudi Arabia and Spain. Sporadic CJD has a similar incidence abroad and the clustering and similar environments are strongly in evidence.

CJD abroad

One of the most renowned and intensive clusters of genetic CJD in the world erupted in Benghazi, Libya during the late 1980s, where incidence rates of CJD ran at a record level of 31.3 cases per million head of population per year amongst the Libyan Jews. This was officially blamed on the Libyan's dietary fetish for eating sheep's eyeballs, which, it was assumed, was the source of the scrapie infection. Yet no outbreaks of scrapie had been recorded in the local sheep and there is no correlation between people who eat scrapie infected meat and CJD.

But an extremely convincing alternative explanation does exist for the cause of this well-documented CJD outbreak in that the US and UK Governments had launched a short series of massive bombing raids against Libya in 1986. This was in retaliation for the Libyan bombings of a German discotheque. The town of Benghazi, with its military academies and alleged storage depots of thousands of tons of sarin (an OP nerve gas), was the main target of these raids. The local population was thus exposed to the massive detonation of a cocktail of munitions during the raids and the sonic shock bursts of the exploding bombs: it is not surprising that the town was shortly to become the centre of a substantial outbreak of CJD.

Probably the highest incidence cluster of sporadic CJD in the USA has occurred in the Staten Island/Long Island area around the intensively used JFK Airport where both the French and UK supersonic transatlantic aeroplanes land – albeit under more stringent noise regulations than those applied in Europe.

The case of vCJD in the small village of Menfi in Sicily was also sited in an area of opencast strontium and celestine quarries and cement production, and next to the former World War II bomber air base at Sciacca. In the first days of July 1943, Sciacca and Menfi endured a sustained aerial bombardment of ordnance during the Allied invasion of Sicily. The US Chemical Corps, which fired white phosphorous and phosgene shells, were also involved in this invasion. BSE and scrapie, which I investigated in Sicily and Sardinia, also involved locations that were sited in areas of celestine and other strontium and barium rich bedrocks. They have been increasingly quarried for the production of cement and gypsum used in the construction of roads and hotels to meet the demands of the fast expanding tourist industry. My analyses confirmed that barium and strontium were elevated in the local ecosystems. Gypsum quarrying and processing is also evident in the vCJD cluster around Queniborough and the CWD cluster around Fort Collins in Colorado.

Another extraordinary case of TSE clustering involved a 60-year-old Italian man, who had CJD, and his pet cat, which had the very rare feline spongiform encephalopathy (FSE). The researchers are reasonably certain that the man and the cat didn't contract their illnesses by eating beef, as the prion strains found in their brains were not those associated with BSE. But interestingly the brain tissue in both cases showed a similar prion strain, which was different from previously reported cases of spongiform encephalopathy. Here again there must surely be a common environmental factor in the house or garden, which has caused the disease in these two cases.

When I was field studying in the Far East I investigated a cluster of CJD in the Fuji valley in Japan. It turned out that there was a factory in the mouth of the valley that had been producing the aluminium-manganese alloy panelling for military bomber aircraft since before World War II. The prevailing wind had dispersed the emissions of manganese particulates all the way up the valley. It was therefore interesting that the temporal-spatial epidemiology of this CJD cluster precisely correlated with both the start dates and distribution of airborne pollutants of this factory. My soil and vegetation analytical data later confirmed this.

Aircraft panelling is central, I think, in the causation of another TSE called kuru, found uniquely in the Fore tribe in Papua, New Guinea. This disease has been officially blamed on cannibalism, but cannibalism has been practised all over New Guinea and in other countries throughout history. The question is: why did kuru only erupt in a tiny pocket of Papua New Guinea in the 1950s?

Intriguingly, some of the Japanese bombers, which were manufactured from the alloy plating produced at the Fuji valley factory, got shot down during World War II over the Papua New Guinea jungles where the Fore tribe lived. There are some reports of kuru before the war, which could probably be attributed to the volcanic area's low copper and high manganese diet. But the disease really erupted in the Fore about five years after the end of the war, which links perfectly with the World War II contamination.

The Fore folk had scavenged these crashed bombers and started moulding the metal panelling of the fuselage into cooking bowls for use over open fires, eating bowls, axes, and other tools. The acidic water of the local area would cause manganese and aluminium to leach out of the metal bowls and into their food, thus providing extra metal intake over and above their previous diet. Perhaps the eating of the brain in their cannibalistic practices exacerbated the problem of manganese contamination, by enabling the manganese (which accumulates in the pituitary gland in the brain) to bio-concentrate. But cannibalism was practised all over New Guinea at that time and, if cannibalism is involved at all, it is probably as a secondary factor. The primary cause as far as I am concerned is the contamination from the panelling of the crashed bombers.

The successful transmission studies on kuru were mostly carried out by the inoculation of homogenate directly into the brains of monkeys. Oral transmission of kuru with homogenate could not be achieved by mouth, but only when the homogenate was introduced directly into the stomach by tube – which is intriguing. What does this first stage of digestion do to arrest the pathogenicity? This scenario does not prove kuru was caused or even spread by cannibalism. Cannibalism was abandoned in the sixties and kuru has almost died out. This could easily be because the initial high-level exposure to contaminants has fallen off dramatically since the forties/fifties and an increasingly western diet has provided balanced mineral intake for the Fore tribe. This closely parallels the demise of lytico-bodig neurodegenerative syndrome in Guam, which I also

investigated. I would only have been convinced that oral transmission had a role if food products, as opposed to homogenate,
consumed by mouth had produced kuru in the experimental work.

The Fore were self-sufficient in their local volcanic copper-
deficient ecosystem, so the manganese contaminant was able to
substitute on vacant copper-protein bonds, such as the prion protein, thereby rendering their brains unable to deal with the intensive sources of low-frequency infrasonic shock in their vicinity, i.e.
the bombs which they had accidentally exploded during the
scavenging sessions on the crashed Japanese bomber aircraft,
which is well documented, as well as the constant earthquake tremors of that area. The Fore live over a major tectonic rift line and
suffer the severe electric thunderstorms of that area — it's a very
'infrasonic intense' environment.

I'm of the opinion that many neurodegenerative diseases are very
closely related and the human TSEs are no exception. Lytigo-bodig
is a neurodegenerative syndrome that arose in Guam at the same
period of history, also in my opinion through contamination events
and a poor nutritional balance of minerals in the traditional diet.
Researchers found that patients with lytico, an ALS-like condition,
often had a small amount of bodig, a Parkinson's-like condition.
There was sometimes evidence of other neurological conditions in
these patients, such as supranuclear palsy and post-encephalitis.
Some researchers had even thought that the prion protein might
turn out to be involved as well. Interestingly there was no real
exclusivity of pathology defining each condition but rather a collage
of various pathologies, which appeared in slightly different patterns
in each patient.

The metals — the talent in the body, after all — lead astray their
dull old solid workhorse partners, the proteins and sugars. The
great potential of metals to do work and to deliver life is in their gift,
but their orbiting electrons need handling with kid gloves. An
analogy might be with the rock star (presumably of the heavy metal
variety) who in the right setting, on stage, really delivers the goods,

but in the wrong setting, when confined to the neat, ordered psychology of the hotel room, his structure is challenged and all hell can break lose.

Silicosis is a lung condition that results from occupational exposure to the dust derived from asbestos sheeting. Intensive investigation by the scientific community has shown that the causal mechanisms that underpin it are the self-perpetuating, progressive free radical generation. The surface of silicon dust can generate silicon-based radicals that lead to the production of the destructive hydroxyl and oxygen radicals, and hydrogen peroxide, which can damage the surrounding cells.

In TSEs I theorized that the silicate crystal initiates a similar type of self-perpetuating disease process that is insidiously operating in the brain tissues. Once the silicate microcrystal is successfully implanted into the tissues of its host it forms a metal-protein crystal template, which unleashes its unique capacity to generate free radicals and to multireplicate itself. It represents the fundamental mechanisms that are common in the natural process of bio-mineralization – the phenomenon known as osteogenesis – which propels the growth and maintenance of the hard tissues, such as bones and teeth throughout the bio-system.

Silica has been shown to act as an essential precursor for osteogenesis in the bone-forming cells, as well as playing a major role in activating the ingenious life generating group of proteoglycan molecules that are involved in the formation of bone, cartilage and other tissue structures throughout the body. It seems that the body harnesses the semiconducting properties of silica as an ingenious means of conducting the electrical signals that activate the formation of the proteoglycan molecules. These play a crucial communicative role in switching on the secretion of various hormone-like growth factors, i.e. nerve growth factor and fibroblast growth factor, which mediate the growth and maintenance of the structural scaffolding that supports a diverse range of tissues throughout the body.

Rudolf Steiner was one of the first people to highlight the crucial role of silicon in the biological system. His realization that silicon provides the important 'basis of growth' represents just one of his many insights into the fundamentals of the living world.

Recent research has identified that high concentrations of silica are present in the mitochondria of bone-forming cells, as well as in the proteoglycan molecules themselves, providing evidence for the importance of the silicon crystal in the processes of tissue generation. The bio-dynamic force of silicon is probably provided by its semiconducting property, which could also account for the diverse functional roles that silicon performs in so many biological processes involved with growth, repair, storage of information, organization, rhythmic response. But much like the electronic properties of any type of crystal, once the silicon crystal is contaminated by minute amounts of impurity, its electrical properties can be altered, to the extent that it can no longer perform its correct biological function.

This ability to manipulate the electronic behaviour of crystals has been deliberately harnessed in the industrial world, where 'doping' of crystalline materials has become a fast expanding high tech science in which crystal materials are specifically tailored to suit highly sophisticated electronic applications. The silicon and other crystals that are present within the natural environment can become tainted following exposure to various natural and man-made forms of pollutant. Once the mammalian body starts to absorb tainted silicates that have bonded with impurities, such as heavy metals and radioactive metals, then it is reasonable to assume that the chronic intake of these contaminated crystals could instigate bio-electrical problems within such electrically sensitive tissues as the brain.

Any minor intrusion at any point along the pathway of bio-mineralization can reap deleterious consequences on the overall strength and durability of the structural framework of tissues that holds the whole organism together. In respect of diseases like TSEs, Alzheimer's disease and asbestosis, the natural process of bio-mineralization has become corrupted as a result of the introduction of these industrially tainted types of silicate pollutant into the tissues. The formation of these tainted silicates is brought about by the bonding of natural silicates in the open environment with metals like barium, strontium, manganese that originate from a variety of sources of industrial or naturally occurring pollution. A more severe class of corruption can result from the incorporation of silicates that have bonded up with radioactive metal species such as strontium, plutonium, thorium, uranium and caesium. This problem can become extremely serious in ecosystems that are rooted in soils naturally high in silicates, i.e. in topsoils that lie over bentonite clays and have been exposed to significant bursts of radioactive fallout.

Once these tainted silicates have breached the body barriers — the blood-brain and blood-nerve barriers — and substitute themselves at the sites where the natural silicates are normally operating, then any body process that is normally regulated by silica will be compromised. Once the rogue silicate microcrystal has implanted itself into the tissues, it is free to seed the bizarre self-perpetuating pathogenic process that has been well demonstrated in the lungs of those unfortunate victims of asbestosis. But the crux of the CJDs seems to pivot on the fact that this aberrant hypermineralization problem has been seeded in the soft tissue regions, such as the brain, instead of the hard tissue regions where it would normally occur. Recent research has shown that the natural forms of aluminium silicate do actually bond with the prion protein, which supports the proposal that silicates are a key causal component in TSEs.

Sheep May Safely Graze

In 1998 I decided to expand my horizons and embark on a refreshing eco-detective trek to analyse the environments around the world in which transmissible spongiform encephalopathies (TSEs) have erupted as high-incidence clusters. By scanning the overall characteristics of each location, I hoped to pinpoint the common causal factors – the aetiological needles in the haystack. There were precedents for this type of approach which had inspired me, particularly the work of scientists such as Carleton Gajdusek and Yoshiro Yase who had travelled to Guam to study mineral profiles in relation to neurodegenerative diseases.

Against a backdrop of flamboyant and sometimes threatening scientific scenery, I researched in some of the exotic and dark regions of Iceland, Slovakia, Calabria, Sardinia, Sicily, Colorado and Japan – areas where an assortment of animals and humans had demonstrated a high incidence of TSE. After many false leads my observations revealed several common toxic denominators – low copper and high levels of some metallic microcrystals, such as manganese, barium, strontium and silver, combined with high intensities of low-frequency infrasonic shock. Many of these factors were associated with military activity or industrial contamination.

It should be pointed out that many metals, such as manganese, copper, strontium and zinc, are essential in very small quantities for animal and plant life and are not toxic per se. For example, the recommended daily allowance for manganese in adult humans is 2.5–5 mg.

I discovered various sources of the microcrystals, from the atmospheric fallout from naturally occurring and industrial sources of combusted manganese oxide from volcanoes, acid rain, steel/

glass/ceramic/dye/munitions factories, lead-free petrol refineries and the take-off airspace beyond airports. Atmospheric manganese, like silver and aluminium, can be absorbed directly into the brain via the highly efficient nasal-olfactory inhaled route, which perhaps enables sufficient concentrations of manganese to build up in the brain and to precipitate disease.

I was also fascinated to discover that TSE affected populations were living in areas that were enduring 'front line' exposure to intensive shock bursts of low frequency infrasound – military and quarry explosions, volcanic and earthquake shocks, low flying supersonic jets and Concorde over-flights.

Another common feature of TSE environments was the Pre-cambrian granite and volcanic mountainous terrain. The high altitudes and higher exposures to ultraviolet light were also interesting and I was curious as to whether photo-oxidative effects might contribute in some way to the disease. It took much research before the full relevance of these additional facets could be integrated into the causal equation.

Iceland

Scrapie is the TSE that affects the brains and nervous system of sheep and goats. The name is derived from one of the symptoms of the condition, in which affected animals will frantically scrape themselves against rocks or fences to relieve the itching. The disease was first identified in 1732 on the Cheviot hills in the UK, where sheep grazed on the lava and ash slopes of the ancient Cheviot volcano. Scrapie is also a problem on my own doorstep along the Brendon Hills in Somerset, where there is a history of manganese and iron mining.

Since 1934 the volcanic island of Iceland has had a major problem with scrapie, or *rida* as it's known there, and consequently it provided an ideal location to start my investigation. In September

1998 I flew to Reykjavik with my brother Nigel to meet the epidemiologist and man in charge of *rida*, Professor Sigurdur Sigurdarson. He kindly drove us around for a couple of days and showed us wild geysers and epic waterfalls, as well as taking us to some *rida* farms to collect samples. For the second part of our trip we flew up north to Akueyri, where some of the most intense scrapie clusters had occurred.

We were sitting in the petrol station café on the edge of the dark and sombre fishing town of Dalvic, having hitched a ride on the post van from Akueyri. Wet and muddy and over-laden with equipment, we slouched up to the counter and ordered two coffees from the proprietor. He pushed a button on a machine and when we asked how much he shook his head — it's free. We felt a twinge of embarrassment as we settled with our wet gear into half a dozen seats in the pristine, white tiled café. We sipped the excellent coffee and gazed into the core of the rain-swept valley. A plateau loomed at its end, veiled in cloud, like Conan Doyle's lost world, and the rain continued. After an hour we packed and, weighed down with freeloading guilt, we coyly nodded thanks to our host and headed off to the edge of the world.

This area is the most interesting of the *rida* locations because of a pair of neighbouring valleys, one which has had *rida* for decades and the other which is *rida* free. Intriguingly, sheep from both valleys freely intermix on the open mountaintops during summertime, discrediting the conventional theory that *rida* is transmitted via animal to animal contact.

We took samples in Svarfadardalur, the *rida* valley, which runs only 15 miles from and parallel to the *rida*-free valley of Horgardalur. The results consistently showed a level of manganese in the grass two-and-a-half times higher than in the *rida*-free valley, and low levels of the radical scavenger metals copper, zinc, iron and selenium, which are crucial components of several enzymes. The high manganese could be related to a number of factors, such as the higher intensity of precipitation, snow cover, and the annual thawed snow run off recorded in the *rida* regions, as well as the soil acidity and waterlogged organic matter of the peat soils, which render manganese more freely available for plant uptake.

There were also sources of intensive infrasound in the *rida* valley, stemming from the earthquakes and earth tremors, which have consistently issued from the major tectonic fault line that runs past the head of the valley (Dalvik was flattened by one such earthquake in 1938).

Whilst the highest international incidence of *rida* in Icelandic sheep could be partly attributed to the high manganese and low copper recorded there, the protracted 23-hour daylight interval of the Arctic summer would provide a photo-oxidative effect, which may be involved in TSEs. The lower elevation of the sun's rays in Iceland, diminished near the North Pole, serve to decrease the overall summertime intensity of UV exposure in that region. The ozone layer is also thinner above Iceland than at the Equator and, furthermore, clinical signs of *rida* are usually first recognized in August, at the end of the summer mountain-grazing period.

The recent fall in *rida* in Iceland must be partly due to the sharp decline in the total number of TSE susceptible sheep due to the Icelandic Government's prolonged *rida* slaughter policies. The fall could also be due to the nearly total switch from hay, which has much higher manganese levels, to silage as winter fodder.

One unexplained geographical characteristic common to TSE cluster areas involves the isolated rural nature of these communities and their position at high altitudes on peaked volcanic, Precambrian, pine-covered mountain ranges that remain snow-covered for the majority of the year. Other examples include the CJD clusters in the High Tatra Mountains of Slovakia, the Calabrian Aspromonte Mountains (adjoining Mount Etna), the Kofu Mountain in Japan, the Highlands of Papua New Guinea, the CWD cluster in deer of the Rocky Mountains in Colorado, the Aragon Mountains in Spain, the Brecon Beacons in the UK, and more recently the Barbagian and Sopramonte Mountains in Sardinia.

A correlation exists between these mountainous localities and the areas where acid rainfall is prevalent. Acid rain unlocks the availability of metals, such as manganese, in food chains. It is also widely recognized that the chronic hypoxia of high-altitude living renders mammals more susceptible to oxidative stress, as well as increasing the permeability of their blood-brain barriers to metals. These environments at high altitude are also naturally challenged by higher levels of UVA radiation, as well as the more potent UVB radiation, which in turn generates high ground levels of tropospheric ozone in the more polluted atmospheres. Both UV and ozone invoke oxidative stress in the body.

I would have liked to have returned to Iceland to test for the wider spread of metals, which I was testing for in my later research, and check out barium, silver and strontium in particular.

Slovakia

After the interesting results from Iceland I set off in September 1999 with my brother to investigate both scrapie and one of the world's most intense clusters of sporadic CJD, in Slovakia. I was curious to find out if the high manganese and low copper profile would emerge again from this environment.

There is an incidence of 1 case per 1000 per annum amongst the residents of a group of neighbouring villages in the Orava region on the western slopes of the High Tatra Mountains. This is more than a thousand times greater than the normal incidence of the disease. There is also a smaller cluster of cases in the south, which centre on the rural village of Poltar. Scrapie is also common in these areas.

The main cluster area was around the villages of Zuberec and Malatina where the local people have lived a largely self-sufficient life, growing their food on allotments surrounding the villages. I took samples for analysis of some of their mainstay foods, such as potatoes, nuts and cabbage. The results demonstrated levels of manganese in excess of the average levels usually associated with these crops, but the levels in the pine needles were ten times higher than in the adjoining CJD-free locality. The concentration of metals in pine needles serves as a good yardstick for assessing the levels of metal contamination of ecosystems and is particularly relevant when assessing the levels of atmospheric metal particulates. Interestingly we discovered there is a popular local dietary custom of using pine needles to make 'syrup' and 'tea'.

The levels of copper, zinc, iron and selenium in these home-grown foods were deficient in the TSE zones and this was further compounded by the excessive levels of calcium in the plants of these zones. High levels of calcium in the diet would exacerbate the already deficient levels of copper by impairing its absorption in the gut, due to calcium mediated pH alterations. The prominent cultivation of the 'high calcium' alfalfa crop in the cluster region in Zuberec would further compound the problems.

Scrapie was first discovered in Slovakia in the Pucov region, which turned out to have the same manganese and copper status as the Icelandic scrapie endemic regions, but it's thought to have existed throughout the whole of the Orava region for many decades.

Our chief contact in Slovakia was Dr Eva Mitrova, an epidemiologist at Bratislava University, who specializes in TSEs. She helped to set up meetings with her colleagues in the regions and gave us some useful background information on CJD and scrapie. Dr Mitrova, who was a great host, treated us to an unusual elevenses of Slovakian beer, dispensed from a huge aluminium barrel, wheeled in by one of her protégés. Several plates of local sponge cakes followed and we spent a pleasant hour sitting round the table in her office sipping the light, tasty beer, studying maps of Orava and discussing copper and protein folding – as you do in Bratislava. On a more serious note, she has identified a genetic risk factor associated with the Slovakian CJD area, but also points to the presence of some hitherto unidentified environmental factor that plays a crucial role in the aetiology of CJD and scrapie in these areas.

We found several local sources of atmospheric contamination, such as a television component plant and two large ferromanganese factories at Siroka and Istebne situated a few kilometres upwind of the main CJD zones in the valley. The problem of atmospheric manganese contamination may have been compounded further by the presence of other ferromanganese plants located to the north, across the Polish border.

In Poltar, the southern CJD area, we found the dominating presence of a large glass factory – manganese is employed in the glass-making process. Some of the CJD victims had been employed in these factories for varying periods of their working lives. People working at or living downwind of these factories would have been exposed to significant levels of airborne manganese and silicates in both the northern and southern CJD area.

The factories were originally constructed during the Communist era at a time when 'green' was definitely not on the agenda and scant resources were channelled into reducing the emissions of toxic pollutants. The emissions from these factories are locally renowned to form clouds of 'smog' which travel up the valleys in a southerly/easterly direction for several kilometres, precisely over the communities where CJD has erupted.

Public fears of atmospheric pollution with manganese dioxide, nickel and other metal compounds had prompted a study in 1995 by the Dolny Kubin Health Institute. They analysed the hair of children for metal levels in the towns of Dolny Kubin, in the Orava CJD cluster region, and Oravska Lesna, where there was no CJD. The results demonstrated 12.945 mg/kg of manganese in the hair of children living in Dolny Kubin and 2.832 mg/kg of manganese in children residing in the CJD-free Oravska Lesna area. Analyses of the other metal levels in the children living in the two regions were normal. The World Health Organization maximum limit for manganese is 4 mg/kg.

The explanation for the high manganese level is that the prevailing westerly winds pick up airborne metal particulates emitted from the factories and carry them the 5–15 miles to the 'rain belt' western foothills of the Tatras, where rain delivers the pollutants back to the ground. The local food and the atmosphere become contaminated and any TSE-susceptible genotypes become at risk of developing the disease.

Whilst a background incidence of CJD is thought to have existed in Orava for many decades, it is interesting that the disease didn't start to rise until the 1950s, with scrapie taking off a few years later, peaking at the high rates encountered in the 1980s. This perhaps reflects a delayed neurotoxic response to the development of the ferromanganese and TV manufacture industry in Orava, and glass production in Poltar. An early life exposure of a copper-deficient individual to a manganese-contaminated environment could lead to the formation of the manganese form of the misfolded prion protein in the CNS, with clinical TSE manifesting many years later in adulthood.

Two CJD cases within a cluster of six cases in Burlington, Ontario, Canada were immigrants who came from the Orava CJD region. Burlington is commonly referred to as 'Steel City' because of the prevalence of steel factories in that vicinity.

Italy

I made two trips to Calabria and Sicily, in the south of Italy, to investigate a sporadic CJD cluster as well as scrapie. Since 1995, 20 cases of CJD have erupted amongst a community of TSE-susceptible Greek-Italian people who live in a hamlet located in the south of Calabria. The victims carry a rare prion point mutation called E200K, which predisposes to CJD, but it is interesting that there are no cases in the many other carriers of this mutation in the wide Greek-Italian diaspora outside the village. This strongly indicates an environmental factor has triggered the disease. The majority of the CJD cases involved part-time small farmers who also worked locally at a railway train and carriage repair factory where arc-welding of manganese enriched steel is carried out. This type of occupation provides an exposure to substantial doses of airborne manganese, where the metal can be absorbed directly into the brain via the nasal-olfactory route. Other CJD victims had worked at a clothing factory where chemical dyes containing manganese and other metals are handled.

The very poor socio-economic status of this Greek-Italian community in the village lead them to eat large quantities of home-grown foods. The soils that I sampled from the CJD victims' gardens demonstrated a high manganese level (71 mg/l) and very low copper (1.7 mg/l). There were three other metals that I found to be raised — strontium at 2.4 ×, barium at 2.8 ×, and silver at 3.8 ×.

The 'bergamot orange', which contains the potent photosensitizer furocoumarin, is also grown in this region. A photosensitizer is a chemical compound, found in food products and the body, which is readily prone to photoexcitation — a process which creates energy that is transferred to other molecules and makes the body more sensitive to light. It's a phenomenon that is exploited to kill cancer cells in photodynamic therapy.

I had noticed the concurrent exposure to high intensities of UV, foodstuffs and synthetic chemicals containing systemic photo-sensitizing molecules in TSE cluster zones. These substances bond to chromophores, such as melanin, forming long-term stable complexes that impair the photoabsorption process, thereby exacerbating the pro-oxidant effects of UV by generating toxic singlet oxygen and/or the superoxide radical.

Since the early 1980s significant amounts of furocoumarin-rich citrus waste, containing the peel fraction, were fed to UK dairy cows — a practice also adopted by all of the other European countries affected with BSE.

Furthermore, the deer and sheep in Slovakia's and Colorado's cluster zones consume large quantities of alfalfa, which can contain high levels of the photosensitizer psoralen. Another TSE-affected species, the nocturnal mink, sometimes received a combined treatment of psoralens and UV for enhancing the pigmentation of their pelts prior to slaughter.

Also relevant are the potent photosensitizers called terpenes, contained in the aromatic atmospheres of the pine forests and in pine needles, which are eaten by the deer and human populations in the Colorado and Slovakian TSE zones respectively.

Another condition related to UV light is photokeratitis or 'snowblindness', which traditionally develops in those who live and work in the snow-clad mountain areas as a result of visual contact with the higher intensities of UV photons reflected from the snow. Higher UV intensities are also encountered in coastal locations where sand and sea reflect the UV rays. The residents of the Calabrian hamlet were moved from their remote mountain village and rehoused by a government-funded scheme in a new coastal settlement. A combination of their newly constructed white painted houses (unique to this area), widespread coastal view and the surrounding bare white sandstone hillside terraces has caused the development of a 'UV hotspot'. UV radiation is also more intense in the broad vicinity around volcanoes where chlorinated emissions have thinned the ozone column in the stratosphere above – thus permitting greater intensities of UV light to penetrate the earth's surface following an eruption.

On my second trip to the area I discovered what may turn out to be the clinching factor in the Calabrian CJD cluster. The residents had been moved out of the mountain village due to the unsanctioned burial and incineration of unexploded ordnance and other toxic wastes close by. This had apparently gone on in the Aspromonte and Barbagian Mountain regions of Calabria and Sardinia, where both the local human and farm animal populations have recently demonstrated an increased incidence of TSEs, Alzheimer's disease and brain tumours since the 1990s.

Collusion between the Mafia and the military was first established after World War II, when the Allied armies had eagerly off-loaded their stockpiles of unused ordnance via many of the Mafia clans operating in Calabria and Sicily at that time. Today the situation hasn't changed much; a network of industrial bodies are covertly paying the Mafia groups a 'cut price' to dispose of a wide array of toxic chemical and radioactive wastes. These are invariably transported to one of the many illicit 'fly tips' in the south of Italy where they are incinerated or dumped directly into mountain ravines or incorporated into building blocks for houses. Calabria plays host to over 400 of these unofficial toxic dumps.

The cases of BSE, scrapie and variant CJD that I investigated in Sicily occurred in locations where celestine and other barium and strontium rich bedrocks have been increasingly quarried for the production of cement and gypsum to meet the demands of the fast expanding tourist industry. My lab analyses confirmed this elevation of barium and strontium. Gypsum quarrying and processing is also evident in the vCJD cluster around Queniborough in the UK, and the CWD cluster around Fort Collins in Colorado.

The TSE zones also lie very close to the incoming and outgoing flight paths serving the large naval and NATO air bases at Sigonella, Camiso and Trampani Bergi on Sicily, thereby providing the source of sonic shock prerequisite for these TSE outbreaks.

Sardinia

Scrapie was first recorded in Sardinia in 1982. Since then it has presented most intensely in the Barbagian Mountain regions in the central island. I had to abandon my first trip to Sardinia when one of the worst floods in recorded memory hit the Taunton area and my car got stuck (and nearly exploded) whilst trying to cross a flooded country lane. Unfortunately I never made it to Stansted and my brother Nigel went on alone, but I returned a couple of years later.

Scrapie flourished in the late eighties and early nineties in classic

TSE territory in the Barbagian Mountains, occurring at Ozieri, Budduso, known as the granite capitol of Sardinia, Orune, Mount Ortobene, Mamoiada, Gavoi, Ollolai, Olzai and Sarule. A study of the map indicates that these locations are arranged as if in the 'gods' of a vast amphitheatre with the focal point of the stage represented by a new plastics factory in Ottana. This type of mountain valley, shaped like a parabola, where the valley mouth opens into the full brunt of the prevailing winds, was also evident in TSE clusters in Iceland, Slovakia, Calabria, Sicily, Colorado and Japan.

Interestingly, certain topographical landforms are predisposed to serving as acoustic beacons or tannoys of amplified infrasound. For instance, parabola-shaped mountain valleys or coastal cliffs can refract and/or channel incoming prevailing infrasonic waves (radiating from windstorms, oceanic waves, low-fly jet aircraft, thunderstorms, explosions, etc.) into wind tunnels so that they converge to form acoustic beacons of concentrated infrasound at certain locations.

The clustering and the continued occurrence of scrapie in the same Sardinian farm locations make it very unlikely that tainted feed or vaccines, which are the favourite causal theories of the Italian authorities, always end up in the same few western Barbagian farms. These farms also have the typical features of world-wide TSE locations. It was interesting that there was virtually no scrapie in the thousands of sheep grazing on the plains of the island.

I proposed that the many cases in the Barbagian Mountains are related to the industrial centre in Ottana, with the large plastics factory being particularly relevant. Firstly the temporal association is strong. The first cases started about five years after the factory was built, which is consistent with a short period for polluting factors to be established and then the incubation of the disease. The orientation also fits this theory and is very similar to the Slovakian CJD situation where the most intense cluster is east of the factory, downwind. The scrapie largely occurs on the western slopes inclined towards the factory and also at high altitudes (approximately 400–800 m above sea level, Mt Ortobene is 1000 m) where precipitation would be more intense. UV and ozone is also more intense at higher altitudes.

Besides the plastics factory there was a large cement factory (now redundant) situated south-east of the city of Sassari at the head of the valley, which leads eastwards to the cluster areas. Cement manufacture is known to be a major source of silicaceous microcrystalline emissions that generate acid rain and metals, such as barium.

In the southern clusters at Assemini and Decimomannu the scrapie occurred a few kilometres to the north-west of the airport and the industrial centre of Cagliari. They occur beneath the low-fly practice zones of the Decimomannu air fleet at the Barbagia Monte and the Capo Della Frasca aerial bomb test range — the latter being 4 km away from Sardinia's single outbreak of BSE at Arborea.

The results of the 43 metals that I tested for in Sardinia were very similar to the results from the other European, Japanese and North American TSE clusters, which indicated that strontium, barium, manganese and silver were increased between two- and threefold.

The results of the study of all these locations also provided additional evidence that these very rare high incidence TSEs often emerge in areas that adjoin military facilities — where munitions have been manufactured, tested, incinerated, stored or dumped in the past. The close proximity of this unique type of facility to these high incidence hotspots suggests that munitions provide the most likely source of metal microcrystal pollutants.

Japan

In Japan, I investigated an excessively high incidence of scrapie in a flock of sheep that had been introduced onto a remote patch of hillside at Obhiro in Hokkaido. Interestingly, all of Japan's five cases of BSE occurred close by in northern Hokkaido. This area had been exclusively occupied by the Japanese military up until the end of World War II and used as an experimental firing range. Furthermore, low-flying Japanese military jets patrol the coastal waters of northern Hokaiddo owing to its closeness to Russian held territory. Numerous animal experiments were also carried out at this site as well, where horses had been deliberately exposed to detonations of various 'undisclosed' munitions. Although I never analysed this cluster area, geochemical sampling of the indigenous obsidian (volcanic glass) derived soils around this cluster has demonstrated consistently elevated levels of barium ranging between 1500 ppm and 4000 ppm.

*

Since most of the evidence points to the fact that spongiform diseases are caused by a combination of genetic and toxic environmental factors, why do the authorities throughout the world continue to handle these diseases as if they stem from highly infectious origins?

There has been little advance in our understanding of scrapie as a non-infectious disease. If science deems it to be so infectious, why has no one designed a proper trial to prove it once and for all and to elucidate the mechanism whereby it spreads? Slaughter still seems to be the only item on the treatment agenda.

In 2003 I visited some farmers at Warren, in the snow-clad Green Mountains of Vermont. Here the USDA had pounced and seized a flock of local pedigree milking sheep from a farm. Their action was based on the assumption that these sheep could be incubating BSE because they had been imported from Europe, where BSE was still found in cattle. No sheep from Europe had ever been shown to display the clinical or neuropathological profile of BSE. Furthermore, none of the imported sheep were displaying these profiles either, which made the USDA strategy totally incomprehensible.

Later that year I also heard how the German authorities annihilated 10,000 healthy sheep on the most flimsy of scientific pretexts and how this was met with almost complacent acceptance. These reports seem to pop up with ever-increasing frequency from all over the globe — annihilation of a herd of water buffalo in Vancouver, flocks of sheep in Sardinia, deer herds across Wisconsin and 400,000 cows in Germany.

If scrapie can be passed on to humans via oral consumption, why have no cases of CJD erupted in Icelandic sheep farmers or indeed other scrapie countries where eating sheep brains has been popular? In fact, Iceland has only had two cases of CJD, and these victims had both come from the scrapie-free district in the far south of the country. Scrapie material has been included in cattle feed since the nineteenth century and cattle have also had direct contact with scrapie sheep for over 200 years, therefore why didn't cattle develop a TSE before 1984?

The repeated failure of the slaughter programmes to totally eradicate the disease clearly indicates that the cause of this disease lies in the particular environment where these animals were pastured. Despite publication in a variety of scientific journals, the authorities and their key advisors are ignoring these findings and are doing their utmost to marginalize those of us who are trying to pursue this line of research.

All of these spongiform diseases require a genetic susceptibility in their causal interplay, but susceptible individuals require an exposure to the toxic environmental factors before the disease develops.

There are a large number of scrapie-susceptible sheep in Australia that never develop the outward symptoms of scrapie. Yet whenever these sheep are exported to countries where scrapie is endemic, symptoms of scrapie invariably break out — presumably because the environmental causal factors are present in these countries whilst remaining absent in Australia.

The picture I see is one of cronyism amongst a handful of politically motivated scientists in the FSA, DEFRA, USDA and the EU.

They are on the payroll of global corporations whose sole interest lies in forcing open a marketplace for their GM arable protein products. They have no interest in making life easy for their competitors – those of us who are trying to make a living out of selling livestock proteins. This perhaps explains why we are seeing so many of these slaughter programmes instigated in our worldwide farming communities.

Becquerels on the Brain

The tropical island of Guam belongs to the Mariana Islands in the western Pacific. It doesn't quite fit the stereotype of an idyllic tropical island untouched by the modern world, being a highly developed strategic US territory popular with Japanese and Korean tourists seeking the many duty-free bargains in the K Mart super-store. Guam also happens to be the focus of one of the most intensive and mysterious clusters of a neurodegenerative syndrome, which has occurred at very high incidence. It has mainly affected the indigenous people known as the Chamorros, who have lived on Guam for about 4000 years.

I first became interested in this cluster after watching a BBC 2 documentary, *Poison in Paradise*, which featured the journey of the writer and neurologist Oliver Sacks to Guam. (He also wrote an account of the various strands of Guam syndrome research in his book *The Island of the Colour-blind and Cycad Island*.) From this moment I was determined to investigate this fascinating island for myself and travelled to Guam in September 2003 to carry out a total environmental analysis of the three neighbouring coastal villages of Umatac, Merizo and Inarajan, where the diseases had clustered.

The syndrome, known locally as lytico-bodig, simultaneously erupted in several well-defined locations across the South Pacific in the late 1940s and 1950s — the Kii peninsula of Japan, west New Guinea, the islands of Rota and Guam, at 50 times the normal incidence. By the 1960s the disease started to decline, and in fact few cases have appeared in any person born after the mid-1950s. The key epidemiological factors suggest that this cluster represents a delayed neuro-toxic reaction to one or more toxic agents introduced into the local environment during the 1940s. There are likely to be some underlying factors, such as the abnormal mineral profile of the disease region that underpins the condition, which can perhaps explain why there were a few cases before the war.

Lytico-bodig is a mixture of amyotrophic lateral sclerosis (ALS), which broadly represents what the Chamorros call lytico, and Parkinsonism, which represents bodig. In most patients there appears to be a blend of the two conditions, with one usually dominating, and the precise neuropathology appears to be almost unique to each case. It has affected a few non-Chamorro residents and has also developed, but with a 10–20 year lag, in some of the Chamorros who emigrated to California.

Dr Sacks's 50-minute documentary concentrated on the possible role of the cycad, a rather innocuous looking miniature palm tree that provides a staple flour product and medicine, called fadang. During the film a resident made what was for me the key observation of the film. In a 30-second sound bite, which had luckily escaped the cutting room floor, Mrs Santos, wife of one of the victims, challenged the 'cycad' dogma, protesting that they had been eating the cycad fruit for centuries – so why the sudden emergence of this crippling disease during the 1950s? She went on, 'My husband's auntie said it was during the American invasion of Guam when they were bombing the waters – there was something in the bomb that was polluting the water. The children at that time were bathing in it and drinking it.' Unfortunately the film didn't take up this illuminating point.

Hocus Cocus

I met many people on Guam and was fortunate that the local mayor, Tony Quinata, gave me lodgings and a conducted tour of the island. After my initial discussions with several of the Chamorros, I found my investigation focusing on two mainland villages, Umatac and Merizo, and on Cocus Island, an eerie elongated islet rising out of the coral reef a couple of miles off shore. In his book, Dr Sacks sums up just how important this cluster zone is in terms of potential medical answers: 'Here in this village, within the span of a few hundred acres, the secret of lytico-bodig must lie. And with it, perhaps, the secret of Alzheimer's disease, Parkinson's disease, ALS, whose varied characteristics it seemed to bring together.' 'Umatac is the Rosetta Stone of neurodegenerative disease, Umatac is the key to them all.' I was very excited by the prospect of trying to decode this environment and researching its history.

On my second evening I attended an enlightening meeting with an ex-serviceman and atomic veteran, Robert Celestial, and his colleagues. Although I was initially suspected of being a 'CIA plant', I convinced him to the contrary and spent the rest of the evening listening intently to Robert's catalogue of nuclear exposure incidents during the clean-up of the US atomic bomb test sites at Bikini atoll. He had subsequently survived a series of grotesque cancers, which had motivated him to devote the rest of his life to campaigning. He handed me the sworn statement of another ex-serviceman, Vancil Sanderson, which offered a plausible explanation for the poor state of the Cocus Island environment.

Vancil had been stationed at the former tiny naval station on Cocus Island, and his statement told how there was a continuous stream of small naval ships entering Cocus lagoon, which lay between the Cocus Island coral reef and the diseased coastal villages on mainland Guam. Disturbingly, these boats had all been involved in monitoring the atomic bomb tests on the atolls between 1946 and 1963. After each detonation they were taken back to Cocus for decontamination of their radioactive fallout.

Acid detergents and sand blasting were used in the decontamination procedure, and the resulting radioactive debris was discharged directly off the decks and into the open sea. The life of the coral reef was subsequently blighted due to the infiltration of the marine food chain with a radioactive cocktail of strontium 90, barium 137 and caesium 137. A high peak of radioactivity was detected in the surface waters around Guam during a radio-ecological study carried out by the University of Washington in 1959.

The naval boats left a toxic legacy of radioactive decay in their wake – a fallout that could last for up to 60 years. More disturbingly, the radioactive alkaline-earth metals that were involved, such as strontium and barium, are readily incorporated into the calcium of the coral beds, since the atomic arrangement of these metals is nearly identical to that of calcium.

Next day I sailed out to the former tropical 'paradise' of Cocus Island, to see for myself and quickly realized that the accounts I had heard were not exaggerated – the coral reef, on the western sector of the island formerly owned by the US Navy, was in very poor condition. It was cankerous and barren, like a derelict moonscape, and there was little evidence of life except for the solitary skeleton of a juvenile crab that appeared to have been frozen 'mid-scuttle' across the top of a coral block. The general ecosystem of this part of the island was also poor with a few patches of sickly looking vegetation.

My inspection of Cocus – albeit 40 years on from the contamination – seemed to confirm the statements made in Vancil Sanderson's report about the blighting of the coral beds. I found that the ratio of sand to coral on the local seabed was still only about 9:1 – clearly abnormal, since reports written before the US Navy's arrival in the late 1940s referred to a blanketing of coral across the Cocus seabed.

I even saw a rusting bulldozer blade, dumped at the top of the old naval section of Cocus beach – a last reminder of the military tackle that used to push contaminated waste into a landfill pocket on the island.

Despite the tropical heat of that afternoon, I felt a slight shiver down my spine as I watched another boatload of innocent young Japanese tourists alighting on the newly developed 'Cocus Island resort'. I wondered whether they would still be as eager to sunbathe on the silvery white sand or water ski around the lagoon if the toxic secrets of the island had been publicly unveiled.

But the danger posed by the decontamination of the boats in Cocus lagoon was concentrated in the period when the highest levels of radioactive contamination existed 50 years ago. This window of toxic exposure precisely fits the model prediction of the researchers who have been studying the origins of this epidemic.

Unfortunately the Chamorros had continued to draw their staple foods from the last remaining morsels of marine life that had survived the toxic contamination. More disturbingly, they continued to pulverize the chunks of local coral into a fine powder for mixing up with the betel nut and papula leaf – a traditional concoction that is habitually chewed for its sedative effects. The Chamorros' unwitting use of the radioactive coral with the betel represents a very concentrated source of strontium 90 contamination.

It seems that the entire epidemic could have been avoided if the local population had been informed of the purpose behind the US military presence on Cocus. Whilst the villagers had watched the USS *Bowditch* naval vessel carrying out a 3000 sonar sounding surveillance of the Cocus seabed, as well as the fleet of vessels that sailed in for decontamination over subsequent years, they knew nothing about the true nature of the operations at the Cocus station.

'Guamogeddon'

With two major US air bases and a nuclear submarine naval base in operation since World War II, the isle of Guam has suffered from more than its fair share of contamination. In fact Guam was christened the 'coconut curtain' during the pre-1962 period when the isle was out of bounds to any foreign visitors who were not approved by the US military.

The Chamorro elders remember the multitude of bombs that were dropped in the bays during the US invasion of Japanese occupied Guam towards the end of World War II. Whilst the US liberation of Guam was unanimously welcomed, one of the downsides of the conquest involved the toxic liberation of barium-based explosives into the marine ecosystem following the detonation of so many bombs. Wherever the warplanes from the US Hornet aircraft carrier were involved in heavy bombardments during June and July 1944, e.g. along the coasts of Guam, Rota Island, Irian Jaya (New Guinea) and Southern Japan – clusters of similar neurodegenerative diseases have subsequently emerged in the latter three locations. And ever since the war, the US Navy has been carting waste munitions that are beyond their expiry date up to the central mountainous backbone of the island and then disposing of them within an extensive spread of sealed off wilderness under military occupation.

Sadly, the former Senator of Guam, Angel L.G. Santos, had only just launched the publication of a major action report on the radioactive contamination of Guam – on behalf of the 'Blue Ribbon Panel Committee' – when he plunged into a rapid attack of a dementia/neurodegenerative wasting condition, which tragically killed him within two months. Hearsay has it that the Senator had been unearthing discarded US ordnance on his own small farm, suggesting that he had become directly contaminated or that he'd been eating his contaminated home-grown fruit and vegetables.

Considering the correlation which exists between the distribution and timing of the cluster of neurodegenerative disease on Guam and the distribution and timing of nuclear contamination, one wonders why all of the teams of US scientists visiting Guam have failed to recognize such an obvious causal association.

There have been many theories on the cause of the Guam syndrome, most of which have come and gone. One theory focused on the slow intoxication of the Chamorro population following the increased consumption of the cycad fruit during the impoverished years when the Japanese occupied Guam in World War II. This theory plumped for a neurotoxic amino acid called betamethylamino-L-alanine (BMAA), which was present in the fruit as the culprit molecule. But cycads were eaten across the entire island of Guam, and in other locations worldwide, and this theory failed to address why the disease had only clustered in the south of the island.

However it was subsequently found that cycads from the disease areas were especially high in BMAA, but experiments failed to demonstrate that BMAA was neurotoxic at a normal 'life' dose. A secondary theory developed out of this idea, which implicated the fact that the Chamorros had also been eating flying foxes, which feed on and crucially bio-concentrate BMAA from the cycad fruit.

Several geochemical studies have already invesigated the correlation between the Guam syndrome area and the volcanic terrain, and most researchers have arrived at the conclusion that an accumulation of manganese and aluminium combined with low levels of calcium and magnesium played a causal role in the syndrome. Conclusions have suggested that chronic dietary deficiency of the calcium and magnesium induced excessive absorption of aluminium and manganese into the nervous system, triggered by the parathyroid gland. The end result was a build-up of and hypersensitivity to the neurotransmitter glutamate, which caused nerve damage and the build-up of neurofibrillary tangles. However, this metal imbalance theory doesn't account for why the diseases suddenly erupted in the 1950s. Nor does it explain the greatly reduced rates of the disease in the north of the island, where levels of the 'incriminated' aluminium and manganese are equally elevated. It also doesn't explain why the incidence of the syndrome is elevated to 'cluster status' on the nearby island of Rota, where the topsoil is based on limestone bedrock, like the relatively 'disease-free' north Guam. The gradual westernization of the Chamarro diet since the 1960s and the consequent balancing of their mineral intake, together with a reduction of the original contamination, may explain why the syndrome is dying out.

A new research team was dispatched recently from the US

Department of the Interior, led by William Miller and Richard Sanzolone, who conducted another full geo-chemical survey around the centre of the cluster. But all of the positive ground gained in their excellent study was blown apart by the bizarre conclusion arrived at in their paper. The authors had plumped for the assumption that Guam syndrome had been caused by another 'natural toxin' – the toxic blooms of blue-green algae, a phenomenon which they had noticed along the estuaries of the three rivers where the three affected villages are sited.

Not long after this study was finished, the natural water supplies to the villages were abruptly terminated and replaced by the mains supply that fed the rest of the island – no reasons given. When the Mayor of Umatac pressed for an explanation, the US authorities supplied him with papers that included a copy of the unpublished paper by Miller, who had made anecdotal reference to the blue-green algae's toxins as the source of the problem. But how could such a circumstantially derived explanation provide a robust basis for cutting off the water? No analysis had been carried out to determine whether this toxin was present in the drinking water. All three villages had in fact been drawing water from the mountain springs and not from the estuary stages of the rivers where the toxic blooms were spotted. One is tempted to believe that this was a cover story for a much more serious contamination of the springs, which could have resulted from the long-term disposal of munitions in the mountains above the villages.

The legacy of radioactive metal contamination

The results of my soil analyses of 46 metals on Guam indicated that levels of calcium and magnesium in all of the vegetation and fruit in the disease regions were consistently low. In contrast, the levels of iron, aluminium, manganese and strontium compounds in the extensive outcrops of red laterite topsoil on the western side of Guam were high. However, the strontium levels were even higher in both the soil and vegetation in the southern disease areas, especially at the former radioactive naval decontamination station on the western tip of Cocus Island, suggesting the possible presence of strontium 90 and 89 isotopes. Strontium levels were also excessively elevated in the coral and shellfish samples drawn from the Umatac coastline. Barium, manganese, aluminium and iron were considerably higher in the vegetation around Umatac and Merizo. Yams contained excessively high levels of iron and aluminium in the south, but most of the other foods had normal metal levels.

The magnetic susceptibility of the soil was elevated fivefold in the disease area. The higher levels of iron, manganese, titanium and nickel-based compounds in these volcanic soils are probably responsible for causing this. Other factors such as the intensity of natural bush fires, the proximity to the coal-fired power plant, World War II napalm bomb assaults and thunder and lightning storms in this part of the island could have been contributory. These phenomena are known to induce thermal or shock induced remnant magnetism. The increase in magnetic susceptibility suggests that the upake of ferroelectric and/or ferrimagnetically ordered metal nanoparticles from these soils into the body could represent a factor that underpins the pathogenesis of Guam syndrome. The progressive substitution of the normal diamagnetic and paramagnetic metal centres in the central nervous system with rogue ferrimagnetic metal nucleators may subsequently seed the multireplication of metal-protein crystal arrays.

Ferrimagnetic metal crystals interact over a million times more strongly with low level 'earth-strength' magnetic fields than diamagnetic or paramagnetic metal crystals. A ferrimagnetically contaminated individual would then be more at risk of developing the syndrome, because of their potential failure to neutralize the emissions of low level magnetic fields from the external and internal environments.

Guam syndrome hypothesis

I hypothesized that once the gut and blood-brain barrier's permeability is impaired there is an increased uptake of the incriminated metals into the magnesium and calcium depleted brain. I had noticed that the Chamorros followed a customary practice of adding large amounts of salt to meals, which would impair the uptake of the already low level of magnesium in their traditional food (sodium disrupts the uptake of magnesium across the gut wall). Once magnesium is deficient in the body, then these rogue radioactive metals, such as strontium 90 or barium, are able to substitute at the vacant magnesium sites on several enzymes, because these metals possess a similar atomic arrangement to magnesium and calcium, thereby disrupting the healthy function of these enzymes. The free radicals generated by the rogue replacement radio-nuclides could then cause mutations. The magnesium activated enzyme glutamine synthetase is less active during magnesium deficiency, with the result that the highly neurotoxic glutamate molecule builds up in the brain, thereby triggering the downward spiral of these types of diseases.

Irrespective of the levels of magnesium in the tissues, exposure to strontium or barium atoms will also lead to a loss of free sulphate in the body, for the reactive forms of these metals are well recognized to couple up with sulphur and thereby starve the nervous system of one of its most crucial structural caretakers – the sulphated glyco-aminoglycan (GAG) heparin molecules. Once deprived of their sulphur co-partners, GAGs will cease to perform their role in the growth and maintenance of the complex infrastructure of neuronal networking and as inhibitors of crystal proliferation.

Interestingly, the loss of GAG activity has been shown to be responsible for the central mechanisms of Alzheimer's, Parkinson's, multiple sclerosis, motor neurone disease and BSE. The co-clustering of these various types of disease in select geographical pockets around the world suggests that all of these conditions share a common early life exposure to ferromagnetic metal-nucleating agents. Individual genetics and the species of metal involved dictate which disease will emerge as a delayed neurotoxic response to these environmental insults.

Whilst it's widely recognized that the toxic mechanism of radioactive contamination is based on the radio-nuclide's ability to initiate free radical chain reactions which damage DNA – causing a wide array of cancers – it is not so widely recognized that these free radicals can also deform the molecular shape of proteins. Once a protein is malformed it can neither perform its proper metabolic function in the body nor be degraded by enzymes at the end of its working life. The resulting 'rogue' proteins accumulate and clump together to form abnormal tombstone features that choke up the neuronal networks. Each condition is marked by its own distinctive 'tombstone' feature such as the neurofibrillary tangle, Lewy body, Bunina body or prion fibril. Neuropathologists actually seek out the type of tombstone in order to diagnose which type of neuro-degeneration disease has occurred, whether Alzheimer's, Parkinson's, motor neurone disease or TSE.

I have written previously about the involvement of rogue metals binding to the prion protein in place of the usual copper atoms, and how this aberrant substitution of metals induces the malformation of the prion protein. But my most recent observations in the TSE cluster ecosystems indicate that these rogue replacement metals could also carry a radioactive component to their atomic armoury, thereby offering a plausible explanation for the virulent, resistant properties of the deformed prion protein and the causal enigma of BSE.

The malformed prion protein becomes much like a Trojan horse that is shuttled around the circadian mediated circuits of the brain carrying its lethal radioactive cargo of metallic missiles on board – a fire power capacity that is capable of detonating a chain reaction of free radical mediated neurodegeneration.

Not that far from Guam, the famous Fore tribe, who thrived in the remote highland region of Papua New Guinea, were supposed to have contracted a type of CJD, called kuru, through their cannibalism. But, in truth, the Fore folk had accidentally exploded bombs whilst scavenging crashed USAF bombers that had been shot down over their territory during World War II. By the 1950s, the survivors had all developed the kuru syndrome. This was the exclusive event that had caused this exclusive outbreak of CJD in Papua New Guinea. Nevertheless, this cluster was blamed on the tribe's cannibalistic practices by US military medical researchers, despite the other 98% of the population across Papua New Guinea, which practise cannibalism in the same way as the Fore, remaining kuru-free.

Having been sceptical of the cannibalistic cause of this cluster, I have always wondered what substances were in the exploding bombs that had exclusively affected that area. My recent analysis of the soil in those highland craters has confirmed my suspicions.

This brought to mind some other field research I had done on radioactive contamination in the USA, at the Fort Collins wildlife facility in Colorado. The disease here was chronic wasting disease (CWD) in deer and I uncovered evidence of radioactive leaks in the facility that occurred just prior to the first occurrence of the disease. I found a series of published studies that recorded in detail the exposure of the deer to plutonium, strontium 90 and caesium 134. During the 1960s/70s, it seems that the entire operation of the Fort Collins wildlife facility was engaged in radiation experiments, which included the direct injection of strontium 90 and caesium 134 into the deer – in order to monitor the biological effects of these compounds.

CWD also erupted in deer grazing across the copper deficient White Sands missile range in the New Mexico desert, which is a tundra terrain of NATO's Cold Lake air weapons range. It also includes the tank shelling range at Camp Wainwright in the Sandhills on the Alberta/Saskatchewan borders. These environments are chronically bombarded by the test firing of similar types of missile and munitions, as well as playing host to the fast expanding oil and gas drilling industry – another major source of natural radioactive metal contamination.

A similar story emerged when I researched the sporadic CJD cluster in a tiny mountain village in Calabria, Italy. The village was abruptly evacuated for no 'apparent' reason during the 1980s. Since 1995, 20 cases of CJD have subsequently erupted amongst the former inhabitants of this village, in which I had also found a radioactive link.

With these cases most of the emphasis has focused on the genetics of the Greek victims and the fact that they carry a prion mutation. However this does not explain the spatio-temporal aetiology of the cluster because there are thousands of carriers of this mutation in the widely spread diaspora, none of whom has developed CJD. Having the mutation does not cause the disease.

The barium necessities

Another neurodegenerative disease to occur on Guam is multiple sclerosis (MS), although it is less widespread than the lytico-bodig syndrome. One of the metals that I had found to be raised in the Guam disease areas was barium, and it was this same metal that I found had contaminated the key MS cluster areas in Saskatchewan, Sardinia, Massachusetts, Colorado and north-east Scotland. I visited all of these locations in the early 2000s and found that barium was consistently elevated in the soil and vegetation. These high levels stemmed from local quarrying for barium ores and the use of barium in paper/foundry/welding/textile/oil and gas well related industries, and also from the use of barium as an atmospheric spray for enhancing and refracting radio waves along military flight paths and missile test ranges.

I proposed that chronic contamination with the reactive types of barium salts could initiate MS by the conjugation of barium with free sulphate, which subsequently deprived the sulphated proteo-glycan molecules of its sulphate co-partner. This disrupts the synthesis of the proteoglycan, which has a crucial role in the sig-nalling pathways that maintain the growth and structural integrity of the part of the nerve that becomes destroyed in MS, the myelin sheath. Barium intoxication also disturbs the sodium–potassium ion pump, which is another key feature of the MS profile.

The co-clustering of various neurodegenerative diseases in these barium-contaminated ecosystems suggests that the pathogenesis of all of these diseases could pivot on a common disruption of the sulphated proteoglycan growth-factor signalling systems.

The barium facts

Barium is a divalent alkaline-earth metal that is naturally present at high levels in certain soil types, oil and coal deposits and sea water. Barium ores are used for many industrial, agricultural and medical applications, and the insoluble barium sulphate is used as a sus-pension in contrast radiography in human and veterinary medicine. The soluble barium salts – acetate, sulphide, carbonate, chloride, hydroxide and nitrate – are highly toxic and used extensively by the military, and in agriculture, paper making, pesticides, rubber, steel and metal alloys, welding rods, paints, leather, fuel additives, TV and electronic components, explosives, atmospheric aerosol sprays for refracting radar and radio waves, cloud seeding weather mod-ification sprays, radar absorbing paints, ceramics, glazes, glues, cement, bricks, drilling mud, dyes, textiles, glass, water purifiers and magnets.

The distribution of MS clusters correlates with the workplaces and environments associated with high levels of barium. The occupational groups identified as the highest risk for the develop-ment of MS include those involved in paper manufacturing, wood processing, leather, metal (especially zinc-related industries), welding, printing, textiles, electronics and agriculture. Barium salts are employed as key ingredients in all of these industries. Simultaneous exposure to the solvents that are also used in these industrial processes would exacerbate the problem of barium exposure by increasing the permeability of the blood-brain barrier, thereby enabling an increased uptake of barium into the brain.

Some MS epidemiological studies have shown that examinations involving X-ray film exposure of the gastro-intestinal tract represent a significant risk for the development of MS. If this is correct then the customary use of barium sulphate in contrast radiography may represent the pertinent causal factor here, rather than the exposure to the actual X-ray itself. Several studies have shown that toxic doses of barium can be absorbed across the gastro-intestinal tract following use of this supposedly insoluble compound in radiography, whilst other cases of barium intoxication have resulted from the accidental use of the more soluble barium carbonate compound in radiography. It is likely that barium would be absorbed considerably more efficiently across the 'leaky' gut membranes of those suffering from an intestinal condition such as Crohn's disease or ulcerative colitis. This class of patient would represent a higher proportion of those being subjected to this type of exploratory radiography.

The highest prevalence of MS has traditionally blighted subsistent rural populations scattered across the Northern Hemisphere in Saskatchewan, Nova Scotia, Iceland, the Orkney Islands, northeastern Scotland, Northern Ireland, Norway, Sweden and Finland. More recently, high incidence MS clusters have started to emerge nearer to the equator in countries like Sardinia. The limestone-based soils of Saskatchewan and Nova Scotia, the Precambrian granites, basalts and mica schists of Iceland, the Faroes, Northern Ireland and Scandinavia, and the old red sandstones of Orkney and north-east Scotland all naturally carry high levels of barium and low levels of 'free' sulphur. In the case of the Sardinian, Canadian and Scottish MS cluster regions, the local geological veins are sufficiently rich in barytes ore to support the mining of barium. Other studies have suggested, without any supporting data, that elevated levels of lead or molybdenum are common to the soil types associated with MS clusters, but the results of my analyses failed to support this finding.

The coastal position of many of the MS-risk populations on the north Atlantic may be associated with their dietary intake of seafood, such as shellfish and molluscs, which are known to bio-concentrate barium to excessive levels. North Atlantic sea water is notoriously high in barium due to the local seabed geology. The additional intensive use of barium-drilling mud in the North Sea oil rig drilling industry, particularly around the coast of north-east Scotland, must have considerably exacerbated the problem of elevated barium in the marine food chain since the 1980s. The customary consumption of whale meat, shellfish and mussels amongst these risk populations could have unwittingly exposed them to excessive bio-concentrations of barium, due to the whale's dietary intake of algae and plankton, which bio-concentrate barium from the surrounding sea water. There was also an exclusive reliance of the UK animal feed industry on the North Sea as its key source of 'fishmeal' protein – a common component of concentrated cattle feeds during the 1980s and 1990s. Such a practice might have played a causal role in the BSE epidemic that emerged in UK bovines, cats and zoo animals during the 1980s and 1990s. TSEs represent one of the other classes of neurodegenerative disease, which exhibit a tendency to co-cluster alongside MS in these barium-contaminated ecosystems.

The military have been billeted near the MS affected communities of the Faroes, Iceland, the Saskatchewan/Alberta borderland, Guam and the Gulf War zones. This could be correlated with the sudden contamination of the local atmospheres following the detonations of barium-based explosives during military conflicts or exercises, or due to other military uses of barium (such as radar ducting aerosols). There are other potential sources of barium exposure in these clusters that involve the proximity of homes, workplaces or water supplies to quarry explosions or the spreading of spent barium-drilling mud across farmland. In Alberta and Saskatchewan I found this waste product of the fast expanding oil and gas well industry was commonly used in the MS areas.

The developed nations are only too keen to brandish the rogue states as irresponsible for their clandestine development of nuclear and chemical weapons. But they are not so keen to open the secret files of their toxic history to answer the public's demands for data on adverse health effects. A substantial number of helpless human and animal populations were subjected to contamination from various sources without their knowledge or consent. The all too powerful politicians and scientific institutions who enacted these atrocities have made certain that they can never be brought to account.

The only difference between the positions of the developed vis-à-vis the undeveloped nations regarding their handling of weapons of mass destruction is that the less sophisticated rogue states have not yet developed a sufficiently watertight infrastructure to keep their various acts of human and ecological barbarism under wraps. On the other hand, the developed nations have been more successful at suppressing their shameful track records and in so doing they have duped their populations with bogus science. They have misdirected us from the cause of so many pollutant-induced modern day ailments onto an assortment of genetic weaknesses, viruses, naturally occurring toxins or, as in the case of BSE, the sheep scrapie agent. It seems that governments and corporations are conjuring up and capitalizing on this phenomenon of 'natural' scapegoats for their own self-protection. It guarantees them exemption from the compensation claims that could occur if the connection between ill health effects and bygone atomic antics and compulsory pesticide policies was ever proved.

If the western governments had permitted the secrets of their atomic backwaters to permeate into the public domain, then we might be a lot further forward in understanding the causes of these neurodegenerative conditions today.

If you can understand the cause of a disease or factors that promote it, then you are better equipped to prevent or cure it.

To the Ends of the Earth

When we think of metal poisoning, lead, mercury and aluminium intoxication invariably springs to mind. But some of the insidious toxic properties of the metal manganese have almost been completely overlooked. Modern health authorities could learn a lesson from the alchemists of the Byzantine era who regarded manganese as the black magic metal whereby the quantum capacity of manganese to absorb light and sound can induce a conversion of this metal from an innocuous to a toxic form.

Small amounts of manganese are essential to human beings (around 5 mg is the RDA) but excessive manganese exposure is considered to cause some neurodegenerative diseases. As part of my quest to identify the original causes of BSE, I had travelled to Groote Eylandt – a once enchanted tropical island in the Gulf of Carpentaria, north-east Australia, where bush lands and forests of stringybarked eucalyptus, pandanus and cypress pine have supported several hunter-gatherer Aboriginal clans. A look at the history of this remote island reveals a mixture of 'heaven and hell' scenarios. Not only does the island's soil play host to extremely high manganese concentrations, but its flamboyant rainforest ecosystems have supported some of the most pure bred Aboriginal clans in Australia today. But as I was soon to learn, the tropical charms of a Groote Eylandt of 'pick-your-own' coconuts and turquoise seas can be deceptive to the uninformed outsider.

I was interested in the emergence of a cluster of mysterious progressive, fatal neurodegenerative diseases (collectively known as Groote syndrome) which had erupted in this remote Aboriginal outback of the northern Australian territories. According to the elders, the problem first developed in the late 1960s after a mining corporation started opencast mining of manganese on the island in the early 1960s. The mining caused a fine black manganese dioxide dust to cloak the precise region of the island where Groote syndrome has now emerged – Angurugu village. But experts, funded by the mining corporation, have not surprisingly told a different story on the origins of this disease.

After the broadcasting of my BBC film *Mad Cows and an Englishman* on ABC Four Corners in Australia, I received correspondence from many people concerned about manganese contamination on Groote Eylandt. One of the most inspiring communications came from Susannah Churchill of Canberra who, unlike your average academic, had actually lived with the Aboriginal folk herself whilst researching for her thesis on this disease. Her manuscript on Groote syndrome makes a refreshingly impartial read. It's a study that combines a lateral mix of cultural, genetic and geo-medical perspectives. I could also strongly relate to her suggestion that Groote syndrome was yet another satellite extension of the famous South Pacific clusters of 'Guam syndrome' – pockets of high manganese/high aluminium terrain where a variety of neurodegenerative diseases resembling Alzheimer's/motor neurone/Parkinson's had burst out at an incidence 50 times above the average.

By an amazing coincidence, the parents of my only Australian friend, Jo Wooding, turned out to have once lived in the same house in Canberra where Susannah had lived. So when Jo next visited her parents in Canberra she was able to pick up a copy of the thesis and deliver it directly to me on her return to London. After reading it, I found myself compelled to visit Groote Eylandt. A year later, I received a welcome donation of £500 from a Canadian reader of the Mid-Atlantic Biodynamic Farming Association's website web forum, which had been promoting my work. This enabled me to raise sufficient money to launch my long awaited investigation into the origins of this mystery cluster.

I found myself incarcerated for 15 hours in the glass terminal of

Dar Es Salam's airport at Brunei whilst waiting for a connection. It was like waiting in a greenhouse and I could do little more than while away the time in the internet café. After failing to retrieve my emails on every single monitor along a row of makeshift computers, I eventually threw in the towel. A junior attendant handed me a huge bill and when I protested he threatened to call the police. He scuttled off and made a series of protracted telephone exchanges with his boss who, after much argument, eventually let me off. I spent the next few hours in the greenhouse reading over my notes and staring through the glass walls. I was constantly aware of the dirty looks coming from the staff of the internet kiosk – perhaps the young lad had lost his commission for the afternoon. The greenhouse got hotter and I just wanted to sprawl out in the shade of the palms opposite the terminal. A mind-bending wave of jet lag suddenly overcame me. However the melatonin 'crash out' took me into a more pleasant dimension as the palms were transformed into a mirage of silvery fronds fanning the humid air.

On the final four hour leg of the flight to Darwin, my illusion of the virtual 'clonelike' beauty of the 'Royal Brunei' hostesses was rapidly shattered when one of them walked up the aisle spraying canisters of pyrethroid insecticide into the intakes of the air circulation system. Within minutes, the whole fuselage was transformed into a gas chamber. Despite being assured of the compliance of these chemicals with the World Health Organization's safety standards, I had perhaps gleaned an explanation for reasons why travel on long haul flights represents one factor for the clinical onset of diseases such as the CFS-like 'aerotoxic syndrome', increasingly common in aircrews. I spent the rest of the flight pondering the possible connection between this disease and the spray treatment and exposure to other similar compounds, which can leak from the lubrication system into the air conditioning system.

At 4 a.m. on a summer morning, I arrived in the half-light at the front gates of the Lalara family home in Darwin. The husband was of Aboriginal blood and used to live and work full time on Groote

Eylandt. The son Daniel emerged bleary eyed from the bungalow to greet me – the first friendly face I'd encountered since leaving my family home in Somerset. After the greetings all I can remember was the whirring of the air conditioning fan as I drifted to sleep for two days in a pathetic state of semi-comatose, jet-lagged haze. The bedroom was dark except for a few shafts of sunlight, which had broken through the blinds. I could just make out Australia beyond.

Jenny, the Caucasian mother of the Lalara family, was struggling to hold down her teaching job whilst keeping her invalid husband and adolescent family together. Jenny's persistent stream of emails to me had been instrumental in convincing me about the serious-ness of the neurological crises on Groote and, more importantly, the need to understand the root cause of this disease. If you can understand the cause, you are in a better position to find a treat-ment or a cure, as well as know how to prevent the disease in the future. Jenny had enlightened me on the serious human suffering of Groote syndrome, which served as a trigger to activate the brilliant academic potential tied up in Susannah's thesis – the combination of perspectives that had persuaded me to travel all this way to Australia.

When I first set eyes on the totally debilitated body of Warren Lalara, I was instantly reassured that my reasons for coming were well grounded. I could see why he had been forced to leave his ancestral island home for the more sophisticated care facilities on the mainland, here at Darwin. In trying to greet me, Warren was unable to rise from the tiled floor. I could sense that the once fit and healthy mineworker, and father of two, felt a bit humiliated on my arrival. His legs were sprawled out, pathetically kicking like a frog on ice. Every muscle and bone in his body was shrunk and wasted to little more than a child's size.

Warren had been dumped by the medics, labelled as one of those suffering from Groote Eylandt syndrome, a supposedly incurable, progressive wasting disease that had officially afflicted those of a single Aboriginal clan who lived in the village of Angurugu on

Groote. The disease had purportedly first erupted some years after the missionaries had persuaded the clan to drop their nomadic way of life and settle down to a more 'civilized', western lifestyle.

A growing group of geneticists is rapidly laying claim to the full ownership and academic rights over this new disease. They have coined the name 'Machado-Joseph's disease', and run a host of sharp-suited symposia set in expensive Florida hotels thousands of miles away from Groote Eylandt — the hotbed of the problem. Meanwhile, a rainforest's worth of condescending letters and documentation has been sent to the Aboriginal elders and missionary bodies urging them to join up with the belief that the Aboriginal 'drunken walking' problems are caused by their 'bad seed'. The alleged weak gene was supposedly first introduced by visiting Macassan sailors who had occasionally interbred with Aboriginal women on the shores of Groote about 300 years ago.

To challenge the genetic dogma on the origins of this disease, I travelled several thousand miles to another isolated area where a cluster of this same ataxic condition exists amongst indigenous folk living on the islands of Flores and Sao Miguel in the Azores archipelago. After drawing a range of environmental samples, I unearthed the same abnormal mineral ratio that I was to find back on Groote Eylandt. In fact, the levels of manganese were so high in the black volcanic terrain of these islands that the mining prospectors have considered it lucrative to mine the metal from the local seabeds.

But this theory leaves many vital questions surrounding the origins of the condition unanswered. Why did Groote syndrome only emerge in the 1960s when the hypothetical 'orgies' of interbreeding took place as long as 300 years ago? Why did the gene not cause the disease for those first 250 years? Why have some strains of this neurodegenerative syndrome also ended up affecting white Caucasian Groote residents, who don't carry the gene — albeit only two or three to date? Why has the disease largely only affected one village community yet failed to erupt in the many other global populations where the Macassans, carrying this same gene, have also sailed and interbred?

That evening, I pushed Warren in his wheelchair to the aeroplane bound for Groote. After some comical difficulties manhandling him up the steep steps to the plane, the hostess helped me belt him in. Warren was going to take me back to his former island home of Angurugu and introduce me to the surviving members of his clan — those still living out their lives in the cluster region of Groote syndrome.

The aeroplane filled up with a strange incongruous mix of passengers — western mining tycoons, an Anglican priest and a pair of first time Aboriginal parents bringing their newborn baby home after a hygienic hospital birth. As the plane began its descent to the island, Warren urgently tried to communicate in a croaking voice (since contracting the disease he could no longer talk properly). He was frantically stubbing at the window with the butt of his clawed hand and managed to get out some protracted enunciation of a word, which sounded like 'u-usheerr'. I guessed that he was referring to 'the crusher' since we were passing over some industrial looking bright lights, which must have been those of the mine's crusher where Warren and his neighbours had worked since the early 1960s.

A slight shiver numbed my enthusiasm for the approaching investigation, as I remembered Jenny's stories about the dramatic changes to Aboriginal life since western culture had imposed its controls — one such legacy involved an upsurge in extreme violence and deviant behavioural psychoses. This seems to have run in tandem with the emergence of Groote Eylandt syndrome. For instance, news had travelled from Groote to the mainland last week, reporting how Angurugu residents had awoken to witness two 'payback' killings where some young lads had cut up two people with machetes.

I had also been warned that the mining corporation might get concerned about my arrival on the island and start harassing me for my permit — a tactic that they all too commonly employ to get potential 'troublemakers' off the island! But Warren had already proposed me to the Aboriginal Land Council and for once I was in possession of the necessary permit to visit a territory. Any potential agitators had no choice but to accept my rightful presence on the island.

Brian and Kathy Massey had come to the airport to meet us. I was shortly to discover that they, along with their small group of Anglican missionaries, represented the only non-Aboriginal body of people who really cared about the demise of the Angurugu community. They'd kindly invited us to stay at their day care centre, and after seeing the gigantic size of the centre in relation to the small size of the village I asked Brian whether the incidence rate of Groote syndrome was increasing. As I suspected, he said that there was a record 30 people out of 900 residents who were currently suspected of suffering from Groote syndrome, and explained why the lack of space in their temporary hospital was a pressing issue.

That evening I prepared to go to sleep in the so-called 'dying house'. Outside the night was an intense black and I sensed the restless ghosts of a community at breaking point. A crocodile was croaking down by the creek and a gunshot echoed from an Aboriginal ghetto across the track. Fruit bats were fidgeting in the pandanus trees outside my room. I thought of Warren's helpless vacant stare and his inescapable isolation, and how his ego and life force had almost been crushed out of him. I drew some comfort from a friendly invitation that I'd had to go 'yamming' in the rainforest with Warren's only surviving sister, Gayangwa, who fortunately has not contracted the disease to date.

I awoke to the sound of the missionary woman's keys opening up the health centre for another day. I stepped out of my room to find the wooden veranda of the mission building virtually covered in mattresses, some of which were already occupied by the frail skeletal figures of people in the advanced stages of some ageing condition — probably some variant of Groote syndrome. There was an angelic looking young baby in a dilapidated pushchair who, according to her carer, was suffering from some 'undefined' neurological disorder. She had apparently been born with the condition. Despite her predicament, she gave me one of those broad Aboriginal smiles as I photographed her.

When I rounded the corner to enter the day room, I surprised one of the younger patients, a 19-year-old girl, who skulked off with an ataxic wobble and tremors breaking out in waves along her limbs. I later heard about the case of a pair of twins, famously known as the Bird Girls, who had been born with this same type of neuro-degenerative ataxic wasting syndrome.

Despite the calming presence of the morning sunlight fluttering across the cycad fronds around the mission building, there was an atmosphere of panic. Their most advanced case, Ernie Lalara, had taken a turn for the worse and was shortly to be rushed off on the next plane bound for Darwin. He needed emergency hospitaliza-tion, because his muscle spasms were becoming so permanent that he could no longer keep his head forward or draw breath. All night, he had been crying out like a wild animal in acute agony.

My anger surged to the extent that I could hardly eat breakfast. These formerly healthy Aboriginal communities had suddenly found themselves blighted with a grotesque new disease which first emerged after they'd been persuaded by the early missionaries to abandon their 'savage' nomadic lifestyle and take up permanent residence in the village of Angurugu. I was preoccupied with the intransigent conclusions of the corporation-controlled 'experts' who were making certain that the cause of this syndrome was conveniently ascribed to Aboriginal genetics.

So what was the real cause of Groote syndrome? For a short period, the missionaries had housed the Aboriginal community at the Emerald River Mission site. But the construction of a secret RAF refuelling base in that part of the rainforest during World War II had caused the mission to move a few miles north in 1942 to what was to become the present-day Angurugu village. The missionaries had feared that the airmen would mess around with 'their' Aboriginal girls. Angurugu was constructed directly on pure manganese dioxide bedrock – a feature that was unique to this area of the island. The Mission set about clearing and cultivating a 50-acre field in order to make the village self-sufficient in vegetables. So the new Aboriginal residents found themselves dependent on a food and water supply which was later analysed and found to contain some of the highest levels of manganese in the world. Furthermore, after the mining company set up their opencast mines next to Angurugu in 1962 – where the Aborigines were recruited to work – the surrounding atmosphere of the village was regularly clouded up with a black manganese oxide dust. With the trees felled and heaps of crushed manganese ore piling up near the village, the resulting fine black dust was frequently blown up to storm force, coating the inside of their open houses.

I was convinced that all of the people here, whether in wheelchairs or sprawled out on the mattresses in front of the Mission, were suffering from some form of manganese intoxication. They closely resembled the patient photos in many neurological publications, which I was carrying in my files. I put these papers down on the Mission table, showing the Aboriginal nursing staff the photos of the sick and debilitated manganese mine workers from India, Chile, China, Morocco and Guam. Since the Aborigines had unquestionably accepted the wisdom of the so-called 'superior' medical experts, that this disease was due to their 'seed', they were amazed to see the words manganese intoxication written beneath these photos – photos that clearly resembled the same condition of the patients they were nursing.

I was also concerned that these Aboriginal victims were perhaps suffering from a form of prion disease – better known as CJD – in conjunction with a more generalized motor neurone/ataxic degeneration. But I kept telling myself that such a suggestion might merely be a product of my own wishful thinking, since I'd come to Groote with the Mission to explore the further associations between manganese and prion diseases. The victims of Groote syndrome did appear to closely resemble the cases of variant CJD that have blighted young teenagers in the UK; their shrunken, stick-insect-like bodies, clawed-back hands, bizarre psychiatric symptoms and howling animal cries all combined to remind me of the grotesque vCJD condition.

It is perhaps no surprise to learn that the Groote Eylandt manganese mines, which supply 25% of the total global manganese demand, supplied a highly concentrated manganese oxide to the livestock and human mineral feed supplement market in Europe. I needed to find out if there had been any significant alterations in the source of manganese supplied to the UK cattle feed market from the early 1980s onwards — immediately prior to the emergence of BSE in the UK. It seems that they had indeed changed from using a manganese sulphate additive to a threefold more concentrated manganese oxide additive.

I had also seen the specialist's report based on some slide sections of brain taken at the post mortem of Warren's brother who had also died of Groote syndrome. Two of the slides had demonstrated the presence of fibrillary features — fibrils are unique to the brain pathology of all that have died of spongiform disease. I had wanted to get hold of the actual slides of these brain sections and view them through an electron microscope to determine if the fibrils are composed of prions. Despite assurances that these slides could be made available to Warren's family, they were never sent.

I met the Aboriginal elder and Warren Lalara's surviving sister, Gayangwa, at the table outside and began running through my questionnaires with them. These were designed to work out the dietary habits, chemical and radiation exposures, occupational histories, etc., of every person with Groote syndrome on the island today. Unfortunately, I was unable to apply the questionnaire to the deceased victims, since Aboriginal spiritual beliefs debar discussion of dead people.

Some common factors started to emerge from my interviews. All victims had originated from Angurugu and had therefore endured virtual lifetime exposure to excessive levels of manganese. Most of the victims had also worked in the mines, and this correlation squared with findings published in the *Lancet* on 30 May 1987 that two out of three brothers from Angurugu had developed Groote syndrome. Both of the affected brothers had worked, without masks, in the manganese-sampling mill of the mine, whereas the disease-free brother had never worked in the mine.

All the victims had been exposed to the sonic shock waves radiating from the explosive blasting at the mines and to synthetic pesticides for controlling cockroaches, mosquitoes and flies in their homes. It seems that these pesticides were applied in a cavalier manner without adhering to the recommended application methods. But having come face to face with some of the giant cockroaches that scanned you with their menacing antennae I had some sympathy with their pest control policies! All the victims had also consumed large quantities of salt in their diet. They had also all eaten locally grown wild foods such as yams, cycads and pandanus, as well as the bats and wallabies (which feed off the cycads).

From my studies of previous mineral analysis projects carried out on the soils, foods and water in this village I had gleaned another abnormal feature of the mineral profile in this region, which involved very low magnesium and calcium levels. I was therefore particularly interested in this Aboriginal fad for spreading excessive amounts of salt over their food, particularly as I'd personally watched them spreading drifts of white salt granules over every meal. Sodium is well known to block the uptake of dietary magnesium across the gut membranes, thereby severely depleting serum magnesium levels.

It is well known that manganese can compete for crucial enzyme activation sites with magnesium. So if magnesium is in short supply, manganese can substitute for magnesium at the active site, subsequently causing a failure to catalyse the activation of various crucial enzymes required for healthy metabolism.

Such is the case for the enzyme glutamine synthetase, where a balance of magnesium and manganese is required for activating this vital enzyme's function to break down glutamate into glutamine in the brain. If the enzyme fails, due to high manganese and a depletion of magnesium in the tissues, then highly neurotoxic levels of glutamate will accumulate in the brain, leading to a progressive neurodegeneration. A pathogenic acceleration of the ageing process ensues, which lies at the heart of many neurodegenerative conditions such as motor neurone disease, Alzheimer's disease, Parkinson's disease and the CJDs. Individual genetic factors dictate the class of neurodegenerative disease that develops.

Interestingly, Susannah Churchill's thesis pointed out that this same high manganese/low magnesium mineral profile has been found in the ecosystems supporting the three main neurodegenerative cluster zones in the South Pacific — Guam, west New Guinea and the Kii peninsular in Japan. These largely self-sufficient populations had been succumbing to neurodegenerative diseases at up to 50 times more than the average global incidence at periods in their history. It seems that Groote Eylandt should be added to this list of cluster regions.

It is also well recognized that high levels of manganese in combination with low levels of magnesium will lead to mutations of genetic material in cells, due to the influence of manganese on enzymes that preside over the structure and metabolism of DNA. An abnormal manganese substitution for magnesium can disrupt the binding of messenger RNA to the ribosome, causing an array of subtle disturbances along the genetic pathways (such as the expansion of the DNA amino acid chain). This could result from a manganese-induced inactivation of ribosomal enzymes, which normally require a specific magnesium co-partner to function properly.

The mechanism of a manganese-induced mutation in the absence of magnesium probably explains one of the key causal factors that characterize Groote syndrome as distinct from other similar neurodegenerative diseases. But the corporate-funded scientists have overlooked the very real possibility of a straightforward environmental induced mutation as the cause of the disease. They have run with the convenient half-truth of this causal story, by blaming the mutation on a faulty gene that has supposedly been handed down through the generations of this Aboriginal clan. Despite their theory gaining virtual universal acceptance, their hypothesis fails to explain the distribution and timing of this disease.

That night I wheeled Warren Lalara back to his room, manoeuvring him inch by inch into his bed. I hesitated for a moment, having considered the potential injuries that my amateur manhandling could bring about. But after gaining confidence from Warren's seemingly happy disposition towards my mode of hand-ling, I soon grew accustomed to my new role as a care worker for the next week.

When I went to bed a few hours later, the nightly rioting of youngsters in the village had just begun. At one time I could hear the Aboriginal kids surrounding my hut and clambering under-neath the raised floor. The disturbances went on all night and were apparently a common occurrence. Horrific violent fighting also broke out from time to time, which in a sense paralleled the sudden unexplained cascades of spasms that occur in the muscles of the Groote syndrome victims themselves.

The missionaries and miners had told me horror stories of hatchets being driven through the skulls of 'payback victims', of spear fights, child torture and women being stripped naked and disembowelled alive with machetes. The village doctor confirmed these stories. She was the one called in to deal with the cases of butchered women. She described how she was always stitching up the guts of Aboriginal women who'd survived these assaults. Whilst Aborigines are renowned for their violence, particularly when it is alcohol induced, it is well recognized that this class of insane, manic behaviour is unique to the Aborigines of Angurugu — a style of violence that was largely unheard of during former nomadic days.

According to the records of the social services, arrests and imprisonment amongst the Aboriginal population at Angurugu are the highest recorded per head of population for anywhere in Australia. I recalled a recent report by Canadian toxicologist John Donaldson, who had personally visited Angurugu during 2001. He referred to an incident in the medical clinic where one individual who got frustrated by the length of the queue had thrown a spear at the nurse. He also cited the observations of the explorer Captain Matthew Flinders who had sailed around Australia's coastline in 1803. Whilst his crew had been generally well received by all of the Aboriginal communities they had met around the Australian coastline, it was a different story when Flinders sailed into the unusual blue-coloured waters of Mud Cod Bay, off Groote Eylandt. The deep blue colour of the water reflected the particularly rich bedrock deposits of manganese, which extend out as a platform beneath the shallow bay at this point on the Groote coastline. Flinders recorded the behaviour of the local Aborigines in the ship's log as follows: 'They come at us very strangely ... sending off their children and women and approaching with spears held in a threatening fashion.'

This brought to mind a mineral analysis study that was carried out on the brains of those impulsive mass murderers who'd been electrocuted on death row in the USA. Their brains showed a hundredfold higher level of manganese than found in the brains of those who'd died of natural causes. There are also studies being conducted in California prisons by a professor of psychiatry, Dr Louis Gottschalk of the University of California. He has found elevated levels of manganese in the hair of criminals convicted for murder, rape and violent crimes. Gottschalk states that 'manganese is a marker for violence'.

Around my hut the screaming and abuse reverberated until about four in the morning. At one time it got so bad that I was convinced a poor young girl was being murdered. Deep down I felt compelled to intervene, but the rational part of my brain told me to hold back — I am a father of eight children back in the UK and self-preservation comes first. Each time I attempted to get to sleep, images of Hieronymous Bosch paintings emerged from my subconscious. The illusion of my newly discovered tropical island retreat where I could sit back and get on with some research had been abruptly shattered.

Next morning there was the usual bustle of ataxic victims and care workers on the veranda and I watched a gang of Aboriginal kids gather and hang out in the clearing by the centre. There wasn't a lot to do.

A clanking pick-up truck pulled up in a cloud of dust in front of the mission, and out stepped Dennis, a Goliath-like character who introduced himself as one of the chiefs of the local mineworkers' Union. He was the sort of guy you'd expect to see bouncing at an LA night club rather than cruising around the outback. But Dennis was a dedicated environmentalist and he'd come to take me on a tour of the mines and surrounding areas in order that I could collect an extensive range of soil and vegetation samples. He was convinced that these neurodegenerative problems could no longer be seen as exclusive to his Aboriginal colleagues since one or two of his white mining colleagues had also died from similar neurodegenerative wasting diseases. Others were just beginning to show the first psychiatric symptoms of what was suspected to be manganese intoxication.

Dennis himself was off work due to problems with gout and cardiac arrhythmia. A build-up of urates in the system causes gout, which can commonly result from a breakdown in the enzymatic regulation of the urea cycle and nitrogen metabolism. Interestingly, chronic manganese intoxication interferes with the enzyme arginase, which plays a crucial role in this cycle. Since arginase is an enzyme that is normally activated by the manganese 2+ form, overall inactivation of the enzyme will occur in circumstances of both manganese deficiency and manganese intoxication when manganese 2+ has been transformed into its 3+ form. Manganese 3+ will fail to activate arginase into its fully operational state. This can occur when people with high manganese levels are simultaneously exposed to devices that emit low frequencies of radiation, which are absorbed by the manganese and consequently cause oxidation of the metal into its 3+ form. Dennis not only lived adjoining a low-frequency radio emitting facility, but he also sat alongside a low-frequency radio phone system hooked up in his work cab.

Dennis was no time waster and I was quickly whisked off in his pick-up to a remote part of the rainforest. After a short detour in which we inspected some intriguing Aboriginal rock art inscribed across the face of sandstone outcrops in the middle of the forest, we arrived at the site of the former Emerald River Mission. I could just pick out a straight track of crumbling concrete overtaken by the stringybarked tea tree boughs, which was obviously the old RAF runway. I allowed my imagination to reflect on some of the tense wartime dramas that must have taken place in this compound during that era. The cycad and prickly pandanus had now reclaimed their territory by establishing a profuse infrastructure of trunk and root.

I stuck my sampling trowel into the former gardens of the Emerald River Mission — now a patch of rejuvenated forest. I was relieved to find that this ground was not as hard as the ground I'd been sampling at the Angurugu Mission, which had almost impenetrable, intensively concentrated manganese pesolites (pebbles). I also noticed that these samples were considerably more lightweight than the soil that I'd drawn back at Angurugu, possibly indicating the lower concentration of manganese in these soils. If the soil analyses turn out to confirm my suspicions of this manganese differential, then this would explain why the neurological problems first began after the Aboriginal clans had moved from the Emerald River Mission into permanent residence at Angurugu — the most intensive manganese hotspot on Groote.

We set off once again into the forest to find Mud Cod Bay — an area of sea coast where Captain Flinders had commented on the unusual hostility of the local Aboriginal clan. As soon as Dennis relaxed back at the wheel, he began to open up over his interests in my whole investigation. He talked about the abrupt psychiatric and neurological demise of some of his co-workers in the mine. A guy called 'Monkey' had started to experience sudden unprovoked fits of rage and aggression, as well as insomnia, tremors, depression, fatigue, cramps and unmotivated crying fits – the textbook symptoms of manganese intoxication.

Monkey was coming to meet me at a party in the mining town of Alyangula that night. He had some interesting analytical data collected from the sampling of his blood, where manganese levels were above the excess limit and magnesium was in the low range. I later came across many more white mine workers who'd discovered exactly the same abnormal mineral profile in their blood. A huge lorry 'train' of manganese passed us on the dirt road. Dennis broke off to tell me that there was '150 tons of manganese shit in there'. He then told yet another strange story about a past 'blast' worker at the mine called Walter – a German character who went around in Bavarian lederhosen. Walter would suddenly fall asleep whilst drilling holes for the explosive charges or, much to the annoyance of his employers, whilst driving the 150-ton train of manganese.

I heard many other tales from the local story book of the miners' village, Alyangula. One told of how poor Walter used to fall asleep whilst peddling his three-wheeled push bike. Not long before he reluctantly had to quit cycling altogether; there had been sightings of him peddling up hills and then a few seconds later descending backwards after he'd fallen asleep. It seems that Walter had also developed other psychiatric traits of manganese intoxication, such as paranoid delusions, whilst he was working in the mine. He had apparently fortified his caravan in Alyangula and even installed surveillance cameras. He was convinced that everyone was about to launch an attack on him. In readiness for such a siege, Walter had rigged up an illegal high-tech radio mast to guarantee a totally independent means of contacting his relatives back in Germany should the great day come. The radio was so high tech that he got into serious trouble one day after accidentally intercepting and screwing up air traffic control at Darwin International Airport 500 miles away.

When the full force of neurological symptoms developed, Walter left the mines. The last reports from the poor guy had trickled back from his deathbed in a hospital down in South Australia. Dennis had tried hard to acquire Walter's medical records from the local Groote health clinic, but they had apparently gone mysteriously missing.

Interestingly, most of the miners who'd become neurologically crippled were not only occupationally exposed to the high levels of manganese ore itself, but were also involved with the drilling and detonation of explosives. Perhaps the well-known association between the physical impact of explosive shock waves and its traumatic impact on the blood-brain barrier had disrupted the body's homeostatic regulation, perhaps resulting in an excessive uptake of manganese and other metals into the brain. Furthermore, manganese is a metal that is known to absorb and form stable bonds with phonons – the units of sound energy. The intensity of sound energy that emanates from explosions is probably sufficient to initiate an actual change in the atomic structure of manganese, causing a change in the magnetic capacity of the metal in such a way that the atoms become permanently magnetized (ferromagnetic) after exposure to external magnetic fields. Normally manganese can only be temporarily magnetized (paramagnetic), e.g. it will loose its magnetic charge after it has been removed from the magnetic field.

My view is that once this strain of ferromagnetic manganese contaminates us, our brains could become like a solar charged battery on continuous charge. External sources of environmental electromagnetic energy, like ultraviolet radiation, may accumulate to high levels in the manganese instead of being conducted along the body's electropathways for our own vital, balanced metabolic needs. Could the factors of combined exposure to both phonon energy and manganese explain a further facet of the causal jigsaw of Groote syndrome?

My questionnaire had demonstrated that all of the victims in the Aboriginal stronghold of Angurugu, whether they worked in the mine or not, had also been exposed to the full force of explosive blasting. For the mine had been operating as close as half a kilometre from the village boundary in the past. One notable 'explosive' event entailed an accidental overblast by the mine's former explosive technician George Baker. He had plugged too much nitroglycerine into a bore shaft in order to deal with an extra hard vein of manganese. The resulting detonation blew the figure of Christ off the crucifix in the Angurugu mission church! The few wealthy Angurugu householders who had glass in their windows had got fed up with replacing endless cracked panes.

We eventually reached Mud Cod Bay, a silvery sea cove where a platform of manganese bedrock stretches some way out beneath the shallow seas. I drew some samples from the manganese-tainted mud, which possessed a curious salinated and sandy matrix. Centuries of rising and falling tides have oxidized and reduced the manganese ores backwards and forwards, distilling them all down to a seabed of pleasant pearl blue. I was sampling here, because it was this stretch of coastline where the Angurugu Aboriginal folk habitually spear crabs and turtles for food. My eyes were straining hard to keep open, since the strong midday sun was glaring directly at us and reflecting off the fine crystalline quartz and silica sand. Every few feet the sun highlighted some attractive chunks of coral and conch shells that lay along the top end of the littoral line.

As we drove off, Dennis enthusiastically introduced me to every detail of the unique ecology of rush grasses, orchids and rhododendron that spanned this last strand of land between the forest and the sea. We crossed a few crocodile tracks and I watched in anticipation of seeing one scrambling across the sand spits to reach the swamps along the forest edge.

Although slightly confused over Dennis's true interests, it had become clear that he was channelling his macho energies into some extremely positive perspectives in life. He was more concerned with a genuine desire to preserve the natural environment than the great majority of ardent environmentalists that you meet. He knew the name of every bird in the rainforest, every fish in the bay, the location of every geological vein on the island. His deep-rooted concern for the health of his co-workers was also highly admirable.

That evening I attended the miners' party where anyone and everyone who had been connected to neurological disease and manganese exposure on Groote had been invited. I finally met Kandy, who had been one of the first people to email me after my BBC film had been broadcast on Australia's ABC Four Corners. She had alerted me to the health problems on Groote, specifically telling me of the case of a white girl, called Maxine, who'd worked for several years in the lab at the mine where she analysed the profiles of black manganese dioxide dust samples. She had unfortunately died in her thirties due to a conveniently 'undefined' inherited neurodegenerative wasting disease, which everyone – except the research scientists – had sworn was identical to the Aboriginal Groote syndrome.

That evening I also heard about the abortive attempt of an ABC film news crew to film a piece that was centred on manganese toxicity on Groote. The Miners' Union had contacted ABC over an issue of 'employers abuse of safety standards' at work, only to find that the aircraft that was bringing the film crew over had been prevented from landing. The mining corporation, which owned virtually every facility and service on the island, had debarred them from landing at 'their' airport – the only airport on the island. The Union hit the roof.

That night I failed to sleep again. The silence of the sunset hours yesterday had been transformed into a hellish night. The mob violence had escalated, reaching its characteristic climax by dawn. A man who was embroiled in a petty feud with his son-in-law had been charging around wielding a machete at anybody or anything that got in his way. The police had just discovered an unconscious and seriously wounded Aboriginal youngster who'd been repeatedly cracked over the head with a shovel, according to bystanders' reports. As is the case with all of these riots, the police usually feel that it's unwise to turn up until the next day, often arriving long after the violence has abated. Wise policy, given that there are only twelve police officers stationed on the island. Back in the days when the police were showing up for every incident, they simply inflamed the riots by their intervention. The officers would usually end up being assaulted with a diverse armoury of spears, machetes, guns and hatchets. The miners had told me that if you intervene – much as I had felt compelled to do the previous evening – you get attacked yourself, not only by the aggressors but also by those victims you are trying to rescue.

A couple of well-travelled Caucasian health workers called Stew and Linda courageously live in a house in the middle of Angurugu. I found it unbelievable that they carry on living there, as they have been forced to confine themselves within a dense fortification of six-tier barbed wire interwoven through a chain-link fence. For good measure the perimeter is guarded by a posse of skulking Dobermans 24 hours a day. Stew told me that Aboriginal communities are reputedly aggressive and that Angurugu is exclusively excessively aggressive. That the village community is by far the most violent in the whole of Australia is demonstrated by the number of violent incidents per head of population. And furthermore, the type of violence here could be classed as a form of psychopathic insanity, particularly when it is exacerbated by alcohol.

'It's explosive,' said Stew, who was only just 20 but built like a tank. 'Your country got into all that namby-pamby, politically correct judgemental criticism of the Duke of Edinburgh associating spears with Aborigines, but he was bloody right. I get a spear tossed at me once a week. You Pommies haven't got a clue. Its frontier stuff out here, buddy.'

I feel that the unique exposure of this village population to an environment that probably carries the highest levels of manganese in the world (150,000 ppm in the manganese bedrock topsoil) has a major part to play in the psychotic behaviour patterns of this community.

Post mortems of the brains of miners who have died of chronic manganese-induced neurodegenerative disorders have revealed widespread loss of the neurotransmitter serotonin receptors. Lack of serotonin has been well recognized to be connected to the cause of outbursts of impulsive, criminally insane, aggressive behaviour – a symptom of the manganese madness syndrome seen in miners the world over. Alcohol consumption is also well known to trigger unprovoked aggression and rage in those who are genetically pre-disposed to low serotonin turnover, illustrating the devastating synergistic scenario of chronic manganese and alcohol exposure. Since serotonin levels are under circadian regulation via the day-light/darkness regulation of melatonin from the pineal gland, the characteristic drop in serotonin levels during the night could explain the somewhat unique cycle of nightime violence and day-time peace in this village.

These eco-toxicological problems are further exacerbated by the complexity of a multitude of subjective, political and vested interest pressures operating in the heart of this community. These influences are so sensitively balanced that the health and well-being of the Angurugu people are often forgotten. Whenever a possible solution to this problem has arisen, one or other of the conflicting interests has invariably stepped in the way and blocked progress. The psycho-neuro problems of Angurugu are consequently escalating to crisis proportions. If this was white, middle-class Britain this type of situation would be soon flagged up as top priority and resources would flood in – it would simply not be tolerated. If no responsible, independent authority steps in to break this deadlock, the village could possibly drift into oblivion. The stalwart presence of the Massey family and the Anglicare mission is the only oasis of hope.

It is imperative that an objective third party steps in to take the reins from the mining corporation. Aboriginal communities have always operated on the extreme of egoless, Buddhist-like, laid-back lines, leaving them totally vulnerable to takeover by any type of invading aggressor. The mining corporation's power base has unwittingly found itself replacing the vacuum of endemic Aboriginal anarchy that has long held sway over this island. Many of the corporation's efforts to integrate with the Aboriginal community have been highly commendable and unique as far as mining company track records go, e.g. employing Aboriginal folk to enact an immediate reforestation of mined land with indigenous saplings. Nevertheless they are not equipped or indeed suitably skilled to deal with the escalating health problems, whether they accepted any culpability or not. It also seems unlikely that the corporation would ever be prepared to accept any level of responsibility for the health effects resulting from excessive airborne manganese, which at the very least has been exacerbated by their mining activities. Manganese dust storms envelop Angurugu during the cyclone season, when the winds whip across the storage heaps of crushed manganese and tailings waste. There is also the impact of sonic shock waves, from the blasting of explosives, on the blood-brain barriers of Angurugu residents.

But there is an increasing reluctance amidst the Aboriginal community, as well as the miners, to publicly admit to the escalating levels of psychotic violence in this community. Furthermore there is an outright denial of any association between the violence and the hefty levels of manganese that have been repeatedly recorded in the soil and atmospheres. The denial also extends to any association between Groote syndrome and manganese exposure, although this is not the case with the poor victims themselves, who seem intuitively to understand the cause of their disease. The problem lies with the fact that the one and only economic pillar of this village is the massive royalties that the Aboriginal community are reaping from the mining corporation for the mining of their land. It has become increasingly convenient for both the mining communities and the Aboriginal authorities to sadly apportion blame for the uncomfortable psycho-neuro problems of their community onto the vagaries of some genetic factor plus alcohol abuse. Some Aborigines have put it down to karmic curses on the particular families affected, which is sadly ironic given that the Lalaras, who are embroiled in Groote syndrome, are perhaps the most highly regarded within the clan for their peaceful qualities.

All studies funded by the mining corporation into the health problems at Angurugu have adopted a judicious selection of the causal factors to be investigated. Instead of considering the overall multifactorial causal jigsaw, their conclusions have invariably only blamed individual genetic susceptibility and alcohol abuse, which are convenient scapegoats considering the commercial interests involved.

Dennis's pick-up truck pulled up in front of the Mission. The Groote victims were already parked up in their wheelchairs on the veranda. Some clearly recognized Dennis from their former days of employment at the mine and were still just about managing to pull a smile of recognition. We had planned to go for another sampling tour into the vast local saltmarsh lagoons, which now and again carve inlets into the hinterland and even penetrate the depths of the rainforest. This region was underpinned by the same vein of manganese bedrock as the village, and the marshes have provided the Angurugu Aborigines with a steady supply of giant mud crabs and mussels.

We followed what seemed to be a tank track through the forest — a well-rutted legacy of too many pick-up trucks during the rainy season. But it was now hard and sun baked and the truck gripped well. Wisps of stringybark vines caught in the windscreen wipers, and I saw the brilliant green flashes of parrots in flight — the flamboyant meteorites of the forest.

We eventually pulled out at the borders of the forest and the broad expanse of saltmarsh opened into full view. I tried to take in the full experience of this curious ecology. The salt crust left by some rather exceptional high tides had covered everything and was presumably responsible for annihilating the last stand of bush vegetation along the front line of the forest. A rough assortment of wiry dead mangrove bushes, which had borne the force of seasonal cyclones and the abrasive action of the sand and salt storms, stood as if abandoned by the spirits.

As we dug for samples, our conversation turned to questioning the mining corporation's perspective on Groote syndrome and how they were wrongly ascribing the problem to genetics. Whilst it is true that it is largely only the Lalara family who have been experiencing the neurological problems of Groote syndrome, neither of us could see how this observation alone was sufficient to demonstrate a genetics-only cause. Dennis made reference to a map of Groote that showed the borders of the original territories of the different Aboriginal clans. This map clearly indicated that the original territory of the Lalara clan precisely encompasses the manganese-enriched eastern area of Groote Eylandt. So even during nomadic times, the Lalara clan would have been hunting and gathering foodstuffs that were almost exclusively grown off the high manganese soils and seabed. Even the crabs and turtles which they eat had got their nourishment from a food chain that was directly dependent on the cracks and crevices of the manganese laterite seashore platform.

I was dropped back at the Mission with my samples, to hear the sad news that Ernie Lalara had just died of Groote syndrome in Darwin Hospital. I had sadly never met the man, since he'd left the Mission the morning I arrived, but nevertheless felt a strong connection with his life.

The place was being rapidly evacuated because Aboriginal people do not believe in occupying the living quarters of a person who has just died. They have to smoke the spirit out before they can return. This is conducted at a ceremony where the deceased's home is surrounded by a ring of dead vegetation, and then set alight to smoulder. I had to rush to get Warren and wheel him off the Mission premises fast. I needed to take him to his surviving sister Gayangwa's house, so that he could join in the family mourning. Warren looked mortified. His eyes were lifeless, fixed in a glazed, vacant stare. I didn't know how to console the guy over the death of his uncle. I felt sure that he was also reflecting on how he would be the next to fall victim to the slowly tightening vice of this grotesque condition.

I left him at the front gate of Gayangwa's house. She had come outside, with an unusual air of silence about her, to take Warren and wheel him the final stretch to the front door. Aboriginal mourning sessions can reach bizarre extremes, at least when you compare them with the inhibited practices of western funeral rites – they smash themselves with stones, often drawing blood.

Back at the Mission building there was a strange silence. No longer did the kiddies' feet rattle the veranda planks or the bouts of screaming and crying waft over from the village. With renewed purpose, I spent the rest of the day alone in the forest digging samples of the indigenous fruits such as the yam, pandanus and cycad, which the Angurugu people had been eating for years. Cycads are symmetrical, squat palm trees – often referred to as 'false palms' or *burrawang* by the Aborigines. Their brown, spherical nuts nestle like eggs in a basket, directly attached to a crownlike structure that is centrally perched on top of the stunted trunk. They were growing out of pockets of soil that penetrated deeply into crevices in the pure manganese bedrock. I suddenly sensed the similarities between this place and the grykes in the limestone pavements thousands of miles back home in the Burren peninsula (western Eire) and felt a surge of homesickness in the pit of my stomach. Restless and agitated I continued gathering handfuls of brittle grasses, drawing blood on some well-concealed thorn barbs. I felt the tension of the people, their anxiety over yet another mysterious death from Groote syndrome where one further member of their finest tribesmen had been inexplicably taken.

My questionnaire of the Groote victims had shown that every person who had contracted this disease had eaten cycad at some stage of their lives. It was customary of Groote Aborigines to cleanse the cycad nuts of a natural poison by caging them in a fast flowing stream for a week or so. After detoxification, the nuts are ground down to make a flour for kneading into a kind of bread dough, which was actually baked in makeshift ovens made of local soil — further manganese contamination!

Interestingly, the unusual custom of cycad consumption had been implicated as part of the cause of the Guam, Kii peninsular and west New Guinea clusters of neurodegenerative diseases in the South Pacific. The native people of these regions had also eaten cycad as part of their staple diet.

The finger was initially pointed at a naturally occurring excitatory amino acid, BMAA, in cycads as the causal agent. But after exhaustive tests most researchers dropped this theory. A second theory focused on the fact that the indigenous people of these regions had also been eating bats, which had been feeding off the cycad fruit. In this way the people were indirectly eating the bio-concentrated toxic ingredient, which the bats had eaten with impunity. Interestingly, the results of my questionnaire had also indicated that the victims of Groote syndrome had all consumed bats and wallabies, which also consumed the 'uncleansed' cycad nuts.

Considering that the Guam cluster areas also share the same high manganese, high aluminium, low magnesium/calcium with Groote Eylandt, I was beginning to wonder whether the cycads in disease regions simply serve as more efficient bio-concentrators of these metals than those in non-disease regions. Perhaps it was the metal constitution of this fruit that represented part of the toxic problem all along — a problem that the early researchers had overlooked. So many avenues needed exploration. After labelling my samples, I went to a bed of wandering thoughts and images. The manganese-veiled moon hung over the rainforest and I felt the moons of a lifetime merge with the timeless stars to which Ernie Lalara had returned.

Next morning, Kandy came to pick me up from the Mission. She was a fair-haired, determined lady who had previously served as the health and safety representative for the miners' union, and had been emailing me for ages since my BBC film was shown on ABC Four Corners. Kandy had lived on Groote with her husband for 20 years, having done the hippy-trail around the world back in the 1970s. Both of them were employed in the mines, and she had become concerned over health issues, particularly since her own blood tests had shown the classic high manganese and low magnesium ratio.

We drove off in Kandy's extraordinary antiquated car, which was a cross between a cowboy taxi and a Brooklyn scrap dealer's van. It had squishy leather upholstered seating and a hypersensitive suspension system which generated a comical volley of bounces, reverberating for several seconds every time the car passed over one of the many potholes on Groote's unmetalled roads. We arrived to meet a group of concerned white women in the local hall of the mining village at Alyangula, many of whom had young children and were connected to the mine in some way. This seemed to be a good opportunity for suggesting the potential importance of magnesium supplementation as prevention against some forms of manganese intoxication – particularly appropriate for the healthy embryogenesis of any foetus conceived on this island. For when magnesium is low and manganese is high, manganese can substitute at the vacant magnesium sites on many crucial enzymes, causing them to become inactivated.

One of the most disturbing consequences of the high manganese/low magnesium ratio in the growing embryo lies with the fact that manganese can induce mutations in genetic material by substituting for the magnesium-activated ribosomal enzymes, thereby producing the mutation underpinning Groote syndrome that is so widely seen in the Aboriginal community only ten miles away at

Angurugu. Whilst Aborigines are undoubtedly more susceptible to this specific mutation due to their genetic and local dietary customs (consumption of manganese-rich yams, pandanus, crabs, etc.), the offspring of the white sector of the mining community might also start to develop these types of mutation in the years to come.

Amazingly, the potential of high-manganese exposure to induce mutations is ironically being exploited for positive uses in pharmacology. In the fight to treat AIDS, manganese is being used to inactivate the magnesium-activated enzyme, reverse transcriptase. This deprives the HIV agent of its ability to make multiple copies of itself, thereby suppressing the disease process.

Kandy took me up to the headquarters of the mine, where I'd been scheduled to take a tour of the operations followed by a meeting with the manager of the mine. One of the union bosses then drove me around the different mine locations to view the techniques of opencast mining – felling trees, blasting, stripping off the upper crust of laterites, mining the black manganese dioxide ore bed, backfilling and finally replanting with new trees. I was highly impressed with the replanted rainforest after the mining operations had been completed. Indigenous saplings were being propagated, planted and maintained by Aboriginal labour until it was certain that the trees had taken root. Apart from the difference in the height of the trees, I was unable to distinguish between the original blocks of rainforest and the blocks that had been replanted after extraction of the ore bed. It was apparent that this mining corporation was not operating like some of the more unethical operators at work in South America and New Guinea.

In the worker's canteen I met up with one of the miners who had been eager to meet me. A few years earlier his wife, Maxine, had died of a motor neurone type disease, apparently identical to the Aboriginal Groote syndrome. She had worked in the mine's laboratory to which I was taken next. The chief chemist showed me the fine powdery samples of jet-black manganese dioxide dust that she had worked with. As these lab workers spent all day analysing the stuff, it was easy to see how Maxine might have endured a significant exposure during her time in the labs. Furthermore, the most efficient route of manganese uptake into the brain is via inhalation; the airborne manganese can be efficiently absorbed via the nasal-olfactory route into the brain.

Whilst it was apparent that the mining company had been doing an impressive job regarding the preservation of the environment and safeguarding some of the socio-economic interests of the Aboriginal community, I did however feel that there was a chronic problem with airborne manganese dust being kicked up. Although the corporation had been attempting to dampen down the dust by spraying water, there were storage heaps and tailings heaps of manganese situated a few hundred metres from the village of Angurugu and some storage heaps around the jetty very close to the mining village of Alyangula. All residents had been complaining of black dust settling inside their houses — even the houses that had air conditioning.

It seems that the problems of this community were fundamentally based on the naturally high concentration of manganese in the bedrock, which was very close to the surface — with all local water and home-grown food supplies being contaminated. But the dust that was being generated by the mining operation had considerably exacerbated the problem. It should be remembered that once manganese is inhaled, like aluminium and silver, etc. it doesn't need to travel to the lungs and cross into the blood — it can be absorbed directly into the brain via the nasal-olfactory tract.

I was ushered into the manager's office and started by cracking a friendly joke about the naturally high concentrations of manganese in the cup of tea he was making me. However, the manager seemed more interested in tape recording every word I was saying. He didn't divulge anything about what they were up to and I even failed to extract a map of the main manganese outcrops on Groote from him. Nonetheless, he seemed to be a reasonable guy who was fresh to the job and genuinely interested in environmental issues surrounding metals — well, whenever his company hat was off.

The manager was also continually referring me to the studies at the Menzies School of Health Research and Royal Darwin Hospital in Darwin, which had been funded by the mining corporation itself. These studies concluded that Groote syndrome was a disease solely linked to the genetics of a specific Aboriginal clan which had interbred with the Macassan sailors, who used to visit Groote for trepang three hundred years ago. If these factors were true, why didn't the disease strike many years ago? And, furthermore, why didn't the disease affect all of those other races around the world where the Macassans had also interbred?

But I kept on reminding myself of Gayangwa Lalara's words of wisdom surrounding the first cases of Groote syndrome. She categorically says that there were no cases of Groote syndrome around when she was a child. The first case was her father, which happened after they had settled full time at Angurugu and after the initial mining explorations had just begun. The Aboriginal elders of Angurugu, Murrabuda and Wurramarrba also confirmed this to me. In fact, the only people who have stated otherwise were the authors of the publications at the Menzies School of Health Research. They had alleged that the Aboriginal authorities had informed them that Groote syndrome had been around as long ago as the eighteenth century. Even if the syndrome had been around prior to the 1960s it seems likely that it was at very low incidence. This would make sense because the less intense exposure to mineral extremes that would have taken place prior to the mining operations and relocating had produced far fewer cases of the disease.

I returned to Angurugu little the wiser. Much of the manganese dioxide from this mine was used in products that were being manufactured all over the world, bricks, steel, aluminium/uranium alloys, dyes, batteries, paint pigments, animal feed minerals and fertilizers – industries whose workforces have been associated with clusters of these same types of neurodegenerative disease.

In the afternoon we went out yamming in the rainforest. The

traditional Aboriginal custom of yamming could almost be likened to a religious ceremony. Parties of woman work the woodlands and track down the particular species of vine that nourishes the edible yam. I felt honoured to be able to push Roseanne, a skeletal 33-year-old victim with a stunningly beautiful face, out to the woods in her wheelchair. Like all Aboriginal people, she just accepts her fate with no self-pity, just a Buddhist-like acceptance of her condition. I secretly wanted to whisk her back to the UK and somehow get her well again. I could feel her pain. A few faded traces of red nail varnish still smudged her nails, as though she had just about given up hope of getting married and living a normal Aboriginal life. The other women brought the crowbars, hatchets and spades for digging and extracting the yams. Gayangwa's nine-year-old grandson scuttled around like a monkey through the mangroves with his machete, pairing back the saplings in order to give a poor tree snake hell.

It was a spiritual and enriching experience working with these people. The younger girls were silently scouting around the forest ground with pickaxes whilst Gayangwa was striding around staring upwards, surveying the tree canopy in order to find the edible yams. I began to wonder how she was not hypnotized by the powerful arcs of sunlight cutting through the stringy vines to the forest floor. Where were those withered vines that bore the crisp, heart-shaped leaves of the edible yam? The breeze caught the leaves and they fluttered a gentle forest mantra. Our grail was proving hard to find and there were many false alarms. Every so often Gayangwa had to break off to scold her grandson who was swinging Tarzan-like across our tracks, clinging onto a plait of tough vines. After about half an hour one of the girls called out in an Aboriginal language. I soon got the gist that she had found a scorched vine, which trailed downwards to the earth, lying beside the roots of a mangrove trunk. After digging with the crowbar and then scratching the soil out with our bare hands, we eventually uncovered the yam lying across the backbone of the manganese bedrock. As we dug around it I became embarrassed by my ineptitude, because I'd already sliced straight through the middle of the tuber – its sap was exuding from the wound. They were merciful and we all roared with laughter.

I was interested in yams, because all of the victims I'd questioned had eaten them in large quantities. Analytical tests already conducted had revealed manganese at excessive levels of 1000 ppm in the yam roots. The women were telling me that the yams would make you itch all over if you ate them uncooked. This made me wonder what other toxic substances could be lurking in their tissues – some allergic photosensitizing agent perhaps? My enthusiasm and desire to investigate this further reminded me of my current total lack of funding and inability to take the research forwards until I had a firm offer of funding. This was very frustrating.

As we left the forest, I could see Roseanne in her wheelchair waiting helplessly at the track side for our return. My anger surged again as I remembered the absurd, irrational and unscientific reasoning behind the British Ministry of Agriculture's rejection of my grant application for a three-year project, which the Minister had invited me to submit in the very public forum of a BBC film. I am confident that this project could have achieved some major discoveries and developments into the causes and prevention of these diseases with perhaps £100K. In their wisdom, however, our Government made a two million pound grant to various 'tame' professors for reassessing their guesstimates of the future incidence dynamics of a vCJD epidemic – an epidemic that thankfully never came. We now know that with their fancy statistical computer modelling the predictions were totally wrong. Why? Because the model flowed from an incorrect causal analysis, i.e. that beef consumption had caused vCJD. What useful purpose did this research study serve apart from teaching us the lesson that you must get the cause correct otherwise these types of statistical projections are worthless?

One of the reviewers of my proposal had misread the number of samples that I'd proposed for each cluster location – by twentyfold less than I had proposed – and accused me of proposing too few samples per cluster location, thereby rejecting my application as scientifically invalid. If this had been true, you could merely increase the number of samples to be taken, surely? But despite my pointing out this major error of the reviewer to the Ministry, they ignored my protest and continued to highlight his review as the key criticism, later even inviting him onto their expert TSE surveillance panel. Their review got worse still by splitting hairs over my use of the term 'slice' of soil when referring to the section of soil that is dug out with the sampling trowel. The irony was one of the reviewers actually asked what the word 'slice' meant, despite the widespread use of this term in the bible of soil sampling guidelines, the instruction book of the Natural Resources Management Ltd (NRM). Perhaps this was new to him. The NRM is the most reputable sampling lab in the UK. Having been falsely accused of not including soil pH and the redox potential in my analyses as well, the Ministry also disapproved of my intention to use small cardboard boxes for holding the soil samples – again betraying their ignorance, because I use NRM standard boxes, which are cardboard.

Well, I suppose I should have learnt my lesson by now that being pedantic is the stock in trade of Ministries and multinational corporations. Inspirational is not a word in their vocabulary. One is likely to have stimulating and lively discussions with them about the suitability of cardboard boxes or the appropriateness of one's language – slice versus sample. How do they have the heart to place this tedious, shallow nit-picking in front of the welfare of these victims? My anger eventually drained out in the heat of the tropical afternoon. Perhaps the high concentrations of manganese were beginning to get to my own serotonin receptors.

I got up at 5 a.m. to be sure of collecting all of Warren's and my baggage and getting us to the plane on time. In the half-light I found Warren trying to crawl helplessly across the veranda to reach his wheelchair. His silhouette reminded me more of an injured stick insect than that of a crawling human. Warren obviously felt deeply humiliated by my arrival at such an embarrassing moment so I laughed to put him at ease, pretending that I had not really noticed his predicament. I then got on with helping him to his feet.

My final hour on the island had come and we were about to return to Darwin. Despite some indirect encounters with the extreme violence of this community, I was feeling saddened at having to leave my new friends.

The airport terminal was little more than an open-sided hut and I was pleased to discover that security wasn't quite as tight and time consuming as I had encountered at Washington Dulles post 9/11, otherwise we would have missed the plane.

Some of the missionaries and the Aboriginal folk were already gathering to say goodbye. I was hoping that they were not building up too many hopes in relation to possible outcomes stemming from my visit. After all, I had not as yet been able to secure access to post mortem brain material from any victim who had died of Groote syndrome. The ball is in the court of the Aboriginal community here, for it is important that they reconsider some of their beliefs over the sanctity of the body after death. If they would permit the release of some brain tissue this would help a lot, as we urgently need to analyse for levels and valencies of metals, antioxidant enzyme activities, ataxin 3 and the prion protein status in order to take this research programme further. If you can obtain evidence of a cause, then you can devise controls, prevention and perhaps cures for this horrendous disease. But up until the present day, all post-mortem tissues have been under the control of the tunnel-visionary genetics-only scientists. They are only really interested in viewing the brain material in respect of confirming a diagnosis of the exotic 'Machado-Josephs' mutation.

Research should consider the multifactorial possibilities that several cell lines, enzymes, proteins or metabolic pathways might need to be simultaneously disrupted in order to bring about a specific disease condition. For example, the dysfunction of the prion protein has been heralded as the 'be all and end all' of the BSE and CJD disease process; the dysfunction of the beta amyloid and tau proteins are considered to lie at the heart of Alzheimer's disease. Now we are being told that the dysfunction of another protein, called ataxin 3, lies at the heart of Groote syndrome. While it is true that the disruption of these specific proteins may well represent a key hallmark of a specific disease process, thereby acting as a useful diagnostic marker for that disease, it is counter-productive to disregard all of the other metabolic disturbances associated with the disease.

Given the diverse range of symptoms and pathological damage involved in Groote syndrome, it seems unwise to attempt to relate all of these complications back to a single mutation in ataxin 3. I feel that a multifactorial causal hypothesis, which jointly implicates manganese intoxication and magnesium deficiency, can account for all of the metabolic disturbances, symptoms and pathology expressed in Groote syndrome victims. This includes the important ataxin 3 mutation.

I had managed to persuade two of the foremost metal and protein analytical labs in the world to look at brain material from deceased Groote victims, opening up possibilities for unravelling the riddle of this disease. I wanted to pinpoint the precise metal imbalance affecting the brains of the sufferers. The researchers were perfectly willing and happy to return all tissues after their microscopic analysis had been carried out.

Despite the indirect monopoly of the mining corporation over all current research programmes investigating the origins of Groote disease, zero progress has been made in respect of the victims' interest. Groote syndrome is increasing at an unprecedented rate. After an initial consultation at the health centre, victims are just sent home to endure a humiliating, slow, protracted death. They are told that there is no cure or treatment. They are abandoned, full stop. If it weren't for the excellent physical and spiritual care offered by the Anglicare Mission in Angurugu, the Aboriginal community would be left with no one other than themselves to care for their victims' interests. One way of resolving the whole problem is to abandon the entire village of Angurugu and resettle the residents a few miles away in a new village sited away from the mining activities and the manganese-rich bedrock. This advice was published in the 1980s but totally ignored.

The other approach is to start treating the victims for manganese intoxication. In collaboration with Warren's wife, I had made several abortive attempts to coerce GPs in Darwin to treat Warren with a course of manganese chelators. Whilst it is unlikely that any chelating treatment could actually reverse Warren's symptoms at such a late stage in the course of the disease, at the very least it is possible that chelators might arrest the disease process. Furthermore, I had provided evidence in the form of published studies of successful chelation therapy with manganese-intoxicated miners. So why is no one prepared to treat Warren?

However, despite the cynical comments from one or two nurses at the medical centre, we managed to get Warren onto daily supplements of magnesium citrate tablets. After three weeks of taking the tablets, Jenny reported that his intensely painful muscle spasms had ceased. This improvement was a godsend to Warren, and had enabled him to start sleeping again through the night, as well as improving the functioning of his digestive tract. So, at the very least, these improvements following magnesium supplementation had indicated that magnesium deficiency could account for some facets of the clinical/biochemical profile of Groote syndrome.

After farewells and the usual absurd problems of manhandling Warren up the steps into the plane, we took off. As we flew over the mine, I could see the giant crusher amidst the black beds of manganese that extended right up to the front line of the rainforest. The bulldozers had been advancing to meet the recent spate of increased orders for manganese dioxide from the West. At the same time I thought of the rising incidence of neurodegenerative diseases around manganese processing industries in the West. How far do the black fruits of this island sow the seeds of madness in our cats and cows, our deer and elk, our mink and goats, our death row murderers or, more importantly, our innocent teenagers with vCJD?

At Darwin I handed Warren back to his partner Jenny, said my goodbyes wondering whether I would ever get to see them again, and took my return flight to the UK. At the X-ray barriers, I cracked a misjudged joke about my samples of manganese tripping the alarms, but the officers weren't amused because manganese oxide is a component of some explosives. Considering the more laid-back approach of the Aussie officials, I took the opportunity of asking the officers at the customs point if they would confirm several reports that had come my way nearly two years ago. These reports had come from UK farmers and vets who had visited Australia, up to six months prior to the official announcement of the outbreak of foot and mouth disease in the UK. They had all reported how they had been exclusively subjected to a thorough disinfecting/cleansing treatment when visiting Australia at that time. Some had questioned officers over the reasons for the cleansing, and one farmer was told how UK livestock farming was sitting on a time bomb, which Australia wanted to avoid. But no more clues were given.

To my surprise, the customs lady answered me openly saying that they had known full well about the foot and mouth disease problem brewing in the UK, well in advance of the date of the official announcement in the UK. She could clearly remember the UK's briefing sheets to them during the autumn of 2000. 'The Pommy Government has always been really good over informing us about impending infectious disease crises. It is the Chinese lot who never bother!'

As I walked onto the plane, I wondered why the British Government had not told their own livestock farmers before any-body else. This would have enabled us all to work cooperatively to prevent the spread of the disease five months earlier than we actually did. I wondered whether this revelation from my Aussie customs informant betrayed the fact that our Pommy Government had no real intention of halting the spread of the foot and mouth disease. But I suppose the devious behaviour of the UK Government towards their own people's interests is part and parcel of the global and European (agenda 2000, etc.) diktat to reduce livestock numbers at whatever cost to make way for the increased consumption of multinational controlled GM soya sources of protein.

On the plane, I engaged with some bulky research papers that I'd collected during my field trip, and set about formulating my own conclusions during the long haul flight home. I read the papers from both sides of the controversy: the excellent pioneering manganese studies on Groote by Mark Florence and John Cawte during the 1970s and 1980s; and then the later studies at the Menzies School of Health Research during the 1990s, which launched the theory of an inherited 'ataxin' mutation as the exclusive cause of the disease and which they had termed 'Machado-Josephs' disease. In one sense, I felt that both were partly right and, in an ideal world, the ideas should have merged to formulate an overall multifactorial conclusion on the cause of this disease.

A few weeks after arriving back in the UK the results of my soil/vegetation and water analyses on Groote came back from the labs. This data completely substantiated the earlier work carried out by Mark Florence and John Cawte, showing that manganese was excessively high and magnesium very low in both the soils and the traditional bush foods of the Aboriginal people of Angurugu. In the batch of soil results, manganese had panned out at an astronomical minimum of 84,196 ppm and a maximum of 216,943 ppm in the soils of the Mission gardens at Angurugu where the Aboriginal people had grown their food. By contrast the manganese levels in the soils back at the Emerald River Mission gardens – where the Aborigines lived before Groote syndrome had emerged – had averaged out at 2081 ppm. Magnesium was very low in the soil of all areas tested on Groote.

The analytical data of the vegetation and foodstuffs was equally compelling. Yams dug from the Groote syndrome area at Angurugu yielded excessive manganese levels at 1351 mg/kg, whilst yams dug from the disease-free area of Bickerton Island yielded just 29 mg/kg.

On top of this, the Aboriginal folk who live in Angurugu are chronically exposed to airborne manganese dust that continually blows across their village as a result of the operations of the adjoining mine.

Iron and aluminium were also high in Angurugu, with yams at 1332 ppm and 629 ppm respectively, whilst their levels only yielded 100 ppm and 49 ppm in the disease-free Bickerton Island.

Interestingly the pandanus and cycad didn't demonstrate particularly high levels of any toxic metal, except a slightly elevated level of lead and zinc in the Angurugu cycads, whilst levels were less in the cycads drawn from disease-free regions. Magnesium was depleted in all bush foods, in all types of vegetation tested.

My own conclusion was beginning to gel. I was convinced it was a combination of manganese intoxication and magnesium deficiency that had caused the mutation as well as many other metabolic complications that were evident in Groote syndrome. In addition, the Aborigines were particularly susceptible to this disease due to some as yet unrecognized genetic weakness, along with the fact that they had thrived off a food chain (yams, crabs, fish, etc.) in an environment that demonstrates excessive levels of manganese and deficiencies of magnesium. Furthermore, Aboriginal people use exorbitant quantities of salt on their food, which further impairs the uptake of magnesium across their gut wall. I just hope that in future the clans get more support and direction from their health professionals.

The Wasting Lands

A Department of Natural Resources' truck kicks up the dust across the drought-ridden canyon, its engines reverberating in an agitated mode. It stops at the main entrance gates to the compound. A wildlife officer gets out and walks to the security point, oblivious to the distant thud of a missile exploding across the range. He's investigating an eruption of chronic wasting disease (CWD) in the White Sands Missile Range, an eerie spread of thousands of acres of US military controlled cactus country that spans the southernmost extremes of the San Andres mountain ridge in New Mexico.

This outbreak is particularly significant in that it represents the first cases of a transmissible spongiform encephalopathy (TSE) disease recorded in a deer herd within the state of New Mexico. Furthermore, the affected herd has been confined within the perimeters of this missile range for several decades.

CWD, which is similar to BSE, was originally identified in the late 1970s as a TSE occurring in deer and elk by the veterinary neuropathologist Professor Beth Williams. The disease could have been endemic at low level for many decades, because any rancher or hunter who had noticed these ailing deer hobbling around had probably put such cases down to premature ageing, poisoning or some 'weakling' wasting condition. But now 7 per cent of the free ranging and captive deer and elk residing along a 100 mile length of the Front Range of the Rocky Mountains in north Colorado and south-east Wyoming have been affected with this disease.

This latest outbreak in a new region provides another serious challenge to the viability of the conventional consensus on the origins of CWD. It has jolted institutionalized 'expertise', bringing into question those veterinarians who have plumped for the assumption that some unconventional 'hyperinfectious' agent is spreading via body to body contact through the deer populations. How did the 'infectious agent' jump the 500 miles from the long-standing CWD hotspot zone in Colorado to the previously CWD-free deer residing within the White Sands Missile Range? The 'experts' were baffled and this latest anomaly was placed on the back-burner.

Before the military occupation White Sands was an industrial centre for the mining of wulfenite ores, which contain the copper-chelating metal molybdenum. There has been an ongoing issue of the accumulation of rogue radioactive metals since the military arrived – the legacy of detonating many and various munitions. Furthermore, White Sands has become a leading world centre for monitoring infrasonic shock bursts from around the globe – not least for monitoring the unique intensity of bursts that are radiated by the explosions of their own missiles. The deer herd has played guinea-pig to an unwitting experiment, which has provided further clues to help crack the causal riddle of spongiform disease.

The Atomic Fawns

In the 1960s and 70s a series of well-planned experiments had been carried out at Fort Collins to monitor the exposure of deer to plutonium, strontium 90 and caesium 134 at every level. The US atomic energy agency and government had funded the Colorado department of wildlife and Colorado State University's department of radiology and radiation biology to do the work. I came across details of these experiments whilst browsing through the vaults of PhD theses stored in the basement of the CSU library. They raised some powerful circumstantial evidence to suggest that radioactive strains of the rogue metals that I had been researching could represent the key causal culprit in the origins of TSEs – most par-ticularly in the new strain, more aggressive TSEs. In fact, the paranoia adopted by the global Establishment towards BSE might be explained by the contents of the PhD documents.

One of the trials involved transporting deer fawns back and forth between the deer pens at the department's Foothills facility at Fort Collins and the plutonium-contaminated pastures of the Rocky Flats nuclear weapons factory at Boulder 60 kilometres away. The objective was to monitor the effects and eco-dynamics of leaked plutonium (and its daughter radionuclides) through the body of the deer and within the general ecosystem. A series of radioactive leaks from rusting barrels that stored plutonium-contaminated oil at the Rocky Flats plant (combined with a fire) had enabled the plutonium and its daughter radionuclides to become airborne, contaminating a wide area of the Colorado section of the Front Range. This area has become the CWD endemic area today.

The peak of contamination was during the 1967–9 seasons when the air sampler detected plutonium as high as 0.35 pCi/m3. A programme of environmental monitoring had picked up significant levels of plutonium as far afield as the Pawnee Butt plains, north-east of Fort Collins, and Roxy Ann Mountain. Disturbingly, the levels of plutonium were higher in the livers of the wild deer that roamed the Cache le Poudre canyon at 0.042 dpm/gm than in the deer that roamed near to Rocky Flats itself (0.033 dpm/gm).

The major biological repercussions of these unique experiments were neither reported nor published until 13 years later, when the 1980 paper by Williams and Young reported on the first ever recorded case in 1967 of CWD in a deer. The delay before publication is mysterious, since most scientists would normally trip over themselves to get important novel discoveries into the academic press. Whilst the authors made no mention of possible causal factors, they stated that the TSE-affected deer were resident at the Fort Collins facility in the very same deer pens that had been involved in these radioactive experiments. It is unlikely that the space/time correlation between these unique radioactive experiments and the emergence of a novel neurodegenerative disease is a coincidence.

The subsequent emergence of CWD in the various other wildlife facilities within the plutonium-contaminated region was probably compounded by the fact that there was frequent importation from Fort Collins of wild deer into these other captive facilities. It is also well known that deer frequently escaped from these facilities into the wild.

Furthermore, on studying a map of the distribution of the nuclear missile silos embedded in the terrain that spans the three corners of south-east Wyoming, north-east Colorado and south-west Nebraska, I found a strong correlation with the current distribution of endemic CWD in the wild deer herd today. CWD has also erupted in deer grazing the tundra terrain of NATO's Cold Lake air weapons range and the sand hills of Camp Wainwright on the Alberta and Saskatchewan borders — areas where similar types of missile and munitions are tested.

There were also other sources of local contamination, such as cement kiln fuels, used by the many cement plants in the area, which utilize low-level nuclear waste materials, car tyres and solvents. There is also the nearby USA's former OP nerve gas production plant 'The Rocky Mountain Arsenal', where 11 million gallons of OP liquid nerve agent has been incinerated to date. Surprisingly, I was offered and took a guided tour of the facility.

Where kiln emissions are concerned, the chimneys of the local cement factory at Lyons, according to a report of 16 December 1992 in the *South West Sage* by John Dougherty, the EPA's division of solid waste made an emergency response on cement kiln dust. They stated that they'd found radioactive plutonium and caesium in the kiln dust at Lyons, and at two other plants near to weapons factories in the USA. The contamination was presumed to be the result of utilizing low-level nuclear waste material from the nearby Rocky Flats weapons plant as fuel for the cement kiln.

On a related note, Dr Randall Crom of the Epidemic Intelligence service of the Arizona Department of Health Services at Phoenix reported that a cluster of six cases of sporadic/familial CJD variants emerged around and at the former Hughes missile plant at Tucson, Arizona between 1980 and 1986. There are some obvious risk factors for TSE in such an environment. The plant was involved in assembling Tomahawk missiles — weapons that contained these same radioactive components. More recently BSE and vCJD cases have emerged in the mammals originating from these very areas where the Tomahawk missiles have been routinely test fired. Three of the six CJD victims, who were diagnosed between 1985 and 1986, were workers at this plant and they had no doubt been working with some of these same radioactive metals. Copper chelating chemicals, such as cuprizone, are invariably employed as propellants in the manufacture of missiles. Interestingly, in the 1970s cuprizone was found to induce a type of non-transmissible spongiform encephalopathy, presumably through chelating copper and thus leaving the prion protein unable to fold into its normal functional shape.

Exposure to both abnormal levels of metals and some radioactive metals seems to explain the emergence of every cluster of TSE that has appeared around the world — such as the tiny Aspromonte mountain village in Calabria, which was abruptly evacuated for no 'apparent' reason during the 1980s. Since 1995, 20 cases of CJD have subsequently erupted amongst the former inhabitants of this village. When I trekked up the rocky road to their former village, I was told of an illegal dumping of radioactive waste on the mountain slopes immediately above the old houses. I knew that I had a feasible explanation for this CJD outbreak.

Despite the long tradition of CWD haunting the Front Range foothills, a surge of near hysteria has struck the official US wildlife departments, whose job it is to preside over CWD. Following in the footsteps of the official furore over mad cow disease in Europe, the US Government has sadly adopted the same unproven hypothesis on the origins of these diseases. They believe TSEs stem from exposure to hyperinfectious 'prions' that are readily transmitted via body to body contact (through saliva, faeces, etc.), or via 'prion' contaminated feed. The deer have been 'blamed' for sharing the same feed troughs, and so have the hunters for carrying the 'infectious' agent around with them from shooting region to region.

The launch of any theory on a new disease invariably attracts a fair degree of healthy challenge. But with TSEs there has been an exception to this rule. For instance, there has been no publicity of the fact that British meat and bone meal (MBM) feed, which was held responsible for the massive BSE epidemic in the UK, has been exported in hundreds of thousands of tons and used to feed cattle herds all over the world since the 1960s. The majority of those countries have never suffered a single case of BSE in their cattle herds to date.

To escape the embarrassment of the outright failure of control measures, the UK Government set about hoodwinking the British public and their foreign interests by creating a second 'reinforced' feed ban in 1996, whereupon convocations of 'non'-investigative journalists swallowed the explanations unchallenged. The explanation for the unaccountable 40,000 cases of BSE born after the ban was the unsubstantiated contamination by micro-amounts of MBM left over in the feed silos getting into cattle feed. It was never proved that any BSE material was present in these silos. It therefore takes micro-amounts of MBM, containing micro, or zero, amounts of BSE prion, to cause the disease, and yet macro-amounts caused no disease when exported previously. They then gave full coverage to the fact that the Government was now banning the inclusion of MBM going into feeds destined for all types of farm livestock. The 1988 ban was subsequently forgotten and conveniently erased from the public memory. But today, many cases of BSE have now emerged that were born after this second 1996 ban.

The hyperinfectious myth is based solely on the fact that TSEs can be transmitted in the laboratory, whereby TSE-affected brain homogenate is injected into unfortunate laboratory animals that subsequently contract TSE. However, these transmission experiments prove nothing in terms of demonstrating whether TSEs are caused by a microbiological infectious agent or not. A central problem at the core of this infectious theory is a chicken and egg scenario. When a new 'infectious' disease appears for the first time, where does the infectious agent come from in the first place?

If a chance mutation in the prion gene of a single animal were invoked to get round this difficulty then you would expect to see a slow spread of the disease through the herd through successive generations, and then eventually to adjacent herds. Firstly this type of disease spread is not seen. Secondly, you would need to scientifically demonstrate the mechanism whereby your proposed transmission occurs, i.e. through saliva, faeces, etc.

If, however, you find a contamination event that occurred a few years prior to the disease appearing, and then you find this scenario repeated at many locations worldwide, I would suggest you have, not proof perhaps, but a pretty good answer to be going on with. Remember Occam's razor.

The success of the lab transmission experiments could just as easily be explained by a highly toxic chemical or metal that had killed the original TSE-diseased animal being transmitted into a secondary host. Once again, this feasible alternative explanation has been ignored.

A global study of the most basic rudiments of the history of TSEs suggests that this disease does not spread via animal to animal contact or via ingestion of the 'infected' by the 'uninfected'. For instance, when I was researching the most intense global hotspot of sheep scrapie in the northernmost Icelandic fjords, I found that the Icelandic sheep farmers had adopted the custom of slaughtering any sheep the moment the first symptoms of scrapie emerged. This tradition had not evolved from any fear of the disease exploding in the sheep population, because scrapie has occurred at a fairly consistent incidence for many years in Iceland. But it was carried out because the hard-pressed farmers thought it best to eat the sheep (brains and all!) before the wasting symptoms of scrapie reduced the poor beast to skin and bones. There was also an annual intermingling during the summer months of the scrapie sheep from scrapie valleys with healthy sheep from non-scrapie regions and yet the disease has never appeared subsequently in the sheep from non-scrapie regions. If scrapie is a hyperinfectious disease why does it not spread to sheep from non-scrapie regions?

A historical study of official government attempts to control both scrapie in Iceland and CWD in Colorado reveals the repeated failure of several wholesale slaughter programmes to wipe out the disease. After the deer and sheep had been culled across the vast tracts of land implicated in these TSE-endemic regions, the fresh livestock introduced after a four-year fallow period started to go down with the disease again. This is because the primary con-taminant cause is still present in that environment.

Disturbingly, it seems that the US authorities have failed to learn from this and are following the footsteps of their European coun-terparts, channelling public funds into renewed slaughter schemes in Colorado and Wisconsin — schemes that are ironically no dif-ferent from those that have already failed. The repeated failure of these trials strongly indicates that the primary cause of this disease lies in the particular environmental contamination where these animals were pastured. An analytical field study of these regions provided me with a golden opportunity to pursue this further.

I travelled to North America on several occasions to research CWD. Whilst collecting samples I found myself dodging rattle-snakes and irate gun-slinging landowners on an exciting trek through the parched, copper-depleted canyons of north-east Colorado and south-east Wyoming. My requests for help were answered by an unusual and diverse bunch of people, such as taxidermists, Hell's Angels, native Americans, hillbillies, veterinary scientists and climatologists.

The CWD-endemic mountain area is Precambrian granite, a classic feature of TSE locations. The flecks of mica and schist in the mountains catch the brilliant sun, and reflect it with great intensity into the eyes. I found the intense sunlight and, more importantly, these specific geo-elements that characterized the granite terrain common to so many TSE regions around the world. Furthermore, this observation virtually guaranteed that my environmental analyses would, once again, come back from the lab showing very low copper.

The only spongiform susceptible species which has failed to go down with the disease in the CWD endemic area was the pronghorn antelope — an indigenous antelope that is well adapted to its centuries-old occupation of Rocky Mountain terrain. The pronghorn can conserve levels of copper and selenium in its body considerably more efficiently than any other species of Cervidae. Perhaps its metabolic predisposition for copper conservation, which the other species do not have, explains why the pronghorn has resisted CWD?

I was not surprised when I heard the news that CWD had been identified in deer living around Mount Horeb in Wisconsin — another copper-deficient granite stronghold, which has withstood the erosive elements over time. But for how long has CWD been around in Wisconsin? The disease may have been there for years, but only just been identified because of the recent surge of political sensitivity and scientific intrigue surrounding it, thereby raising 'CWD awareness'. But if CWD has only just emerged, copper deficiency has blighted this granite terrain for centuries and cannot therefore be the sole cause for the recent eruption of CWD. Plain copper deficiency creates its own symptoms in mammals and is clearly separate from TSE, and under normal circumstances does not progress to a TSE.

Colorado

During my first and second field surveys in Colorado I took herbage samples from an 80-mile cross section of the CWD cluster zone; the analysis consistently showed excessive levels of calcium and low levels of copper. On one trip, however, the level of manganese recorded in the herbage and soil was low, probably because it was drawn during the drought conditions of July 1998, which renders manganese less available. However, the soil sampling I carried out the previous October in 1997, which followed a period of rain and snow, recorded considerably higher levels of manganese, averaging out at 317 mg/kg from the same test locations. It is possible that the recent increase in acid rainfall occurring along the CWD section of the Front Range during the winter rain and snow season is also assisting an increased uptake of available manganese from the soil into the herbage. The levels of twelve other metals were normal at all locations tested.

Interestingly, local ranchers in the CWD zone consider that the increased incidence of CWD correlates with the increase in population density of deer and elk in the Rocky Mountain National Park region – the centre of the CWD cluster. Some studies have also confirmed this observation. The ranchers also report an increase in the consumption of pine needles by deer and elk in the over-populated region. The deer have progressively switched to this abnormal substitute ration since competition for the limited supplies of normal foods has increased. The pine needles, particularly in the acid rain-belt districts, contained very high concentrations of manganese, ranging between 214 and 5810 ppm. This may explain why some studies have indicated that CWD is more prevalent in dense herds – the competition for normal herbage is too great and more deer are forced to eat the needles.

The reduced pasture had also caused the deer accidentally to consume far larger quantities of soil than usual – with an increased intake of the metals present in that local topsoil. The veterinary pathologists at Fort Collins University confirmed that increased amounts of soil and grit had been found in the guts of the CWD-affected deer carcasses brought to them for analysis. The carcasses from deer that had died of natural causes did not demonstrate this unusual finding. I had also noticed that many of the CWD-affected deer had congregated to drink around an outsource pond from a water purification plant. They were found to have large quantities of sand and grit in the gut – silver is the most usual biocide in these purification plants and metals are also known to concentrate in these outfalls.

Another, more disturbing issue surrounding manganese intake by the deer stemmed from the fact that hunters were being sold minerals that were intended to attract deer to their hunting territory. The hunters have been unwittingly shooting their own industry in the foot by putting down these dual purpose minerals, which are addictive and force the sturdy growth of the deer's antlers – manganese is the mineral added to force antler growth. My contacts from Wisconsin also reported the use of these manganese minerals in their CWD hotspot region.

When I returned to the area in 2003 I had decided to test for a much wider spread of metals. High costs had previously restricted the number I could test for. I also decided to test metal levels in the deer's antlers, which are recognized to provide a good benchmark for metal status. Because of the history of the sites, I'd also wanted to test for radioactive isotopes of strontium, but unfortunately my purse couldn't stretch to the £100 a test.

When the tests came back they again confirmed low copper levels. Interestingly, I was getting very high levels of three metals that I hadn't tested for before – silver, barium and strontium – in the antlers, soils and pastures of the deer in the CWD cluster zones compared with the areas where CWD and other TSEs haven't been reported. Manganese was again excessive at 2000 ppm in the pine needles.

I think the likely sources of the raised silver, barium and strontium are both natural geochemical and artificial. Silver or barium crystal nuclei are used for aerial spraying or 'cloud seeding' to promote rain in these drought prone areas of North America. Silver is also slightly raised in these soils and was added to concentrated feed pellets.

In addition barium ions are discharged in jet flight paths, in low flight practice zones and around the munitions production and storage of guided missile testing facilities as a means of enhancing and refracting radar and radio signal communications. Barium and strontium are also naturally high and copper and sulphur are low in the dolomite limestone and Cambrian granite/mica schist soil types in these disease zones. Sulphur can bond up with strontium and barium, protecting against toxicity of the minerals.

Spent barium-drilling mud from the local oil and gas well industry has been spread across some of these pasturelands contributing further to barium overload. Metals such as barium and strontium have subsequently bioconcentrated up the food chain and into the mammals, which are dependent on the local copper and sulphur-deficient ecosystems.

I hypothesized in my paper that silver, barium and strontium might be replacing and binding at the vacant copper and zinc regions on the prion protein and on a glycoprotein called the sulphated proteoglycan, in the same way as I had previously noticed with manganese. This rogue metal binding would impair the capacity of the brain to protect itself against incoming shockbursts of sound and light energy. Silver, barium and strontium chelate free sulphur within the body, inhibiting the synthesis of the sulphur-dependent proteoglycans, which results in the overall collapse of the copper-mediated conduction of electric signals along the prion-proteoglycan signalling pathways. This in turn leads to a disruption of the inhibitory currents at the nerve synapses and endplates of the auditory and circadian regulated circuitry, and disrupts the signalling systems that maintain the structural integrity of the nervous system. The resulting silver, barium, strontium or manganese based compounds seed piezoelectric crystals, which incorporate the prion and the iron protein ferritin into their structure. These ferrimagnetically ordered crystals multireplicate and choke up the prion-proteoglycan conduits of electrical conduction throughout the central nervous system.

The second stage of the disease comes into play when the pressure energy from incoming shock bursts of low frequency acoustic waves from low-flying jets, explosions, earthquakes are absorbed by the rogue 'piezoelectric' crystals. The mechanical pressure energy is converted into electrical energy, which accumulates in the crystal-prion-ferritin aggregates (the fibrils) until a point of 'saturation polarization' is reached. Magnetic fields are generated on the crystal surface, which then initiate chain reactions of free radical mediated spongiform neurodegeneration in the surrounding tissues. Since silver, barium, strontium or manganese based piezoelectric crystals are highly heat resistant and carry a magnetic field inducing pathogenic capacity, I proposed that these ferroelectric crystal pollutants represent the pathogenic agents that initiate TSE. They are of course transmissible in some experimental conditions, i.e. by inoculation of contaminated homogenate.

The CWD-endemic region of Colorado is also well noted for its high intensity of natural radiation of low-frequency infrasound. It lies along a major fault line that runs up the Front Range ridge. The area has suffered from mini-earthquakes and tremors over the years, but several publications have highlighted the high intensity of infrasound that derives from the atmospheric turbulence and winds passing over the mountain ridges of this specific region. The intensive quarry blasting activities in this area as well as the intensive testing of missiles at White Sands and another testing range near Mount Horeb serve as sources of artificial infrasound in these recently declared CWD zones.

An alteration in the normal molecular shape of the prion has been shown to be critical to the development of TSEs, indicating that some loss of function of this protein is all part and parcel of the TSE disease process. The prion needs copper to fold correctly and I have hypothesized that the copper found attached to the prion plays a role in conducting the electromagnetic energy from incoming sources of ultraviolet, geomagnetic and infrasonic radiation from the external environment. These energies are utilized for the host's own balanced metabolism for regulating circadian mediated functions, such as immune defence, the growth and repair of cells, sleep-and-wake cycles.

When copper levels are low in the brain, due to certain environmental influences, the prion protein is capable of bonding onto alternative metals, such as manganese, barium or silver. But these foreign substitutes may not act in the best interests of the organism. For instance, manganese will store up electrical energy instead of conducting it, thereby blocking the flow of electro-magnetic energy which is required for regulating certain vital body functions.

One of the properties of manganese is that it can absorb the energy of sound − such as the high intensities of 'phonon' energy, which are radiated in an inaudible low frequency range, known as infrasound. But manganese can only absorb this energy when found in its 'trivalent' 3+ manganese form. The sound energy alters the atomic structure of the manganese so that it can become permanently magnetized. When an individual is carrying excessive levels of this trivalent manganese in his brain and enters an external magnetic field, the manganese bonded prion proteins become permanently magnetized, causing chain reactions of free radical mediated neurodegeneration and TSE pathogenesis ensues.

High intensities of trivalent manganese may be manufactured in the brain by incoming ultraviolet radiation or other eco-oxidants, causing divalent manganese 2+ to lose an electron (oxidative transformation). It is also possible that an exclusive source of trivalent manganese has entered the food chains in TSE-endemic areas. This may be via the incorporation of manganese 3+ into animal feeds or mineral licks, or via their natural presence in the indigenous geological bedrock of the TSE region. Such a scenario may explain why hunters who are eating deer shot in CWD regions, which have thrived off mineral licks and pine needles containing trivalent manganese, will in turn become contaminated with trivalent manganese themselves. These individuals are now susceptible to the low-frequency infrasonic shocks in their hunting environment. (e.g. natural infrasound, rifle shots, etc.).

Not only has this abnormal mineral imbalance been identified in all of the ecosystems blighted by clusters of TSE, but studies at Case Western University have identified a tenfold higher level of manganese and 50% reduction of copper in CJD brains. Furthermore, Dr David Brown at Cambridge University in the UK has produced the TSE-like malformed prion protein in cell culture experiments after adding manganese to copper-deprived cells.

Whilst it is true that all types of TSE require components of genetic susceptibility in their causal interplay, the TSE-susceptible individual needs the additional exposure to these toxic environmental factors before the disease can manifest itself. There are a large number of scrapie-susceptible sheep that live in scrapie-free Australia, but they never develop the outward symptoms of scrapie. Whenever Aussie sheep are exported to countries where scrapie is endemic, symptoms of scrapie invariably break out – presumably because the environmental causal factors are absent in their native Australia yet fully present in the importing countries.

A political perspective

Since so much evidence points to the fact that TSEs are caused by a combination of genetic and toxic environmental factors, why do the authorities throughout the world continue to handle these diseases as if they stem from some undefined and unproven, highly infectious origin? I can only assume that the rigid adherence of Establishment bodies to this line, regardless of whatever new evidence comes to light, merely betrays the current global agenda to depopulate livestock numbers for reasons that have nothing whatsoever to do with health risks to the human race.

The picture is one of a handful of politically associated scientists who predominate in the UK's and the EU's agricultural and scientific ministries. They are either on the payroll of the global corporations, whose main interest lies in forcing open a market for their GM arable protein products, or their labs are often supported by these corporations.

The multinationals are capitalizing on scare stories, which maintain that 'BSE prions will exterminate us all', and they are spinning the propagandist myths that beef, lamb, venison, game and organic food (grown from animal manure) are contaminated with prions and are therefore unfit for human consumption.

We must remain aware that these corporations have invested billions in researching and developing GM arable protein crops and the complementary package of pesticides to go with them. They have bought up swathes of dirt-cheap arable land across Eastern Europe, the Third World and North/South America, and they are clearly going to attempt to quash anyone competing for 'their' protein market.

A basic study of the history of CWD demonstrates that this disease does not originate from deer-to-deer contact. However, the recent discovery of another cluster of CWD in Wisconsin has invoked an official overreaction – a wholesale slaughter policy has been drawn up throughout CWD-endemic regions across the USA.

This latest turn towards a unilateral policy of 'totalitarian overkill' of a few thousand healthy deer has been received with almost complacent acceptance across the country. These perverse and senseless 'carry-ons' have sadly become the daily 'non-stories' of modern times, particularly here in Europe where reports pop up with ever-increasing frequency: the slaughter of a herd of water buffalo in Vancouver, of flocks of sheep from Vermont, Sardinia and thousands of sheep flocks in Germany, the slaughter of 400,000 cows in Germany – all healthy animals. So what next, the slaughter of the entire BSE-free British sheep flock on the grounds that BSE might just appear in British sheep?

The sad twist to this tale is that straightforward copper supplementation of deer in CWD risk areas may be all that is required to prevent manganese, silver or barium replacing the depleted copper at the critical prion protein bonding sites in the deer's brain. This would protect the deer against factors likely to promote CWD such as infrasound and the intense UV light of these mountains.

The Road to Syracuse

When I heard about the senseless slaughter of a flock of pedigree milking sheep in Warren, Vermont, an opportunity presented itself to combine an investigative journey with a short lecture tour and a family holiday.

It was off-season, flights were very cheap and we snapped up the offer of free accommodation in Warren. The visit was organized by John and Devo Barkhausen, who worked locally as furniture makers and public radio show hosts. They came across my work through a friend and thinking I might be able to help contacted me because they were so incensed by the way USDA had pounced and slaughtered the sheep.

By the time we arrived in Boston we were very tired, having travelled from Somerset the previous day with five children in tow. We rented a large car and travelled north. Fortunately the children perked up when they discovered we'd rented a car that actually stopped and started on the turning of a key and the operating of a pedal (unlike our car at home). There were countless other novelties to keep the little darlings amused, such as the experience of cup holders, air conditioning, tinted electric windows and a proper sound system that played CDs rather than chewed up audio tapes. If only we'd known how easily they could be pleased.

Our first stop was in Cornish, New Hampshire at a contact of mine called Suzanne Lupien, who bravely opened her house to us all. The whole trip really owed its existence to Suzanne, who'd distributed one of my articles at a meeting about the sheep issue in Warren. Devo Barkhausen picked it up, read it, and said 'this makes sense' and she and John got in contact with me. We had an amazing dinner and were joined by the cats, who mucked in, one seeming to take a special liking to my helping. For pudding there was possibly the biggest apple pie in the world, topped with thick cream, which was soon scoffed by the cats, with our children not far behind. After a comfortable night we drove out of New Hampshire and on to snowy Vermont, where the weather started deteriorating rapidly. All but the major roads were covered in snow and ice, but the authorities are good at gritting and unlike in Britain our car managed well with the extreme conditions.

We had arranged to meet John at the Warren village store so that he could guide us along the treacherous track to our rooms deep in the forest. As we carefully drove on to the huge and almost empty store car park, a man starting shrieking at us — something about how to park correctly. It was difficult to interpret his frenetic diatribe, but I gather we had apparently failed miserably to observe the niceties of the local parking code, and although we pleaded ignorance of By-law 761/38, the man, seemingly incensed by our Boston plates, told us to 'get back to the city'. It was the only unfriendly voice we heard in our entire time in New England, everyone else being warm and trusting.

As we followed John's car along the narrow lane we glimpsed an extraordinary higgledy-piggledy house through the pine trees, which soon had the children in fits of laughter — until they realized that it was to be their home for the next week.

The international community condo was designed and constructed by a group of radical students of architecture back in the 1960s. The heart of this curious network of straggling apartments was a huge wood fired furnace, which was virtually the size of a room. It was built to take trees rather than logs, and I wondered what the residents would have made of the wimpish British Aga let alone our meagre Rayburn at home on the farm. Anyway when we ended up barricaded in by snowdrifts it provided a ferocious and welcoming heat during our stay.

John and Devo were wonderful hosts. The first night they invited some friends round for dinner and we enjoyed a convivial New

England night of food, drink, conversation and music with their session band.

Next day we drove across the mountains to the attractive town of Middlebury. No one had told us that the mountain road is closed for most of the winter, but despite some heavy snow we made it. First stop was the University of Vermont's Morgan horse farm, and despite the bitter conditions and the fact they weren't really expecting visitors the manager took time to talk to our 'horse mad' teenage daughters, which left us free to wander around the stud. After sampling the local cafés and bookshops in town we drove home very slowly the long way round into what was fast becoming a total white-out.

We ended up snowbound for several days, which prompted the children to try some sledding. For the first time they were really able to enjoy a winter without endless days of wind and rain. Despite temperatures of $-20°C$, which had me huddled indoors, they seemed totally unphased by the cold – but that's children for you.

We took several walks into the forest where I easily slipped into the midwinter silence of the January afternoons. As we walked by the frozen river, we followed our shadows in its mirrored surface. A solitary owl squinted across at us from the brittle icy boughs of a maple tree. Occasionally the peace was shattered by an agitated raven, which flapped off squawking into the forest. It was out here that I found the space to start thinking again.

I gave my first lecture, based on my theory, at the East Warren Schoolhouse, to a small group of local people who I think were persuaded by at least part of my theory. Next day I did my radio interview with John on his show *Politics and Science* at WGDR, Montpelier about the sheep slaughter and its relationship with my theory. The station manager made a big deal of it and took pictures of us, which John told me was unprecedented! The callers were interested in my theories and perhaps were persuaded that agencies such as the USDA are basically a tool of the industries they pur- portedly regulate. After all, they'd experienced first hand the

USDA's illogical destruction of the healthy Friesian milking sheep at the Faillace's farm.

The children were spared this and went off with Margaret for a guided tour of Ben and Jerry's ice cream factory. The highlight for them was meeting a woman whose job for the last 16 years had been to remove random tubs of ice cream from the assembly line, slice them in half without even removing the lids, and sample them. The whole question of sampling ice cream was not lost on our children and this may have had something to do with their choice of things to do that afternoon. We spent another evening feasting – an appropriate pastime in such cold weather I kept telling myself – at the house of some new friends, the Simpsons. The children, true to form, immediately gravitated towards some pizza, stuffing themselves full and finishing it all, only to find that they had polished off all the starters. They can be very embarrassing at times.

I finally gave into family pressure and was persuaded to try my hand at cross-country skiing. In retrospect this was definitely a set-up because I was literally the fall guy. All the children took to skiing really well and I actually thought that I wasn't too bad. At one point, when I took a fall, two of my daughters, Holly and Aster went quickly on ahead to avoid the deep shame of seeing me remove my skis and proceed on foot down a gentle slope and be overtaken by a bunch of three-year-olds. OK, so they were young, but they'd done it before. I was fairly old, unfit and a beginner. Where's the shame in taking it easy!

The USDA's motive for the hopeless slaughter of the local sheep was entirely emotive. Their action wasn't based on good science but on the assumption that these sheep could be incubating BSE because they had been imported from Europe, where BSE was still found in cattle. This was strange because no single sheep from Europe had ever been shown to display the clinical or neuro-pathological profile of BSE. Furthermore, none of the imported sheep in Warren were displaying these profiles either, which made this multi-million-dollar USDA operation seem like a public relations exercise and political statement, rather than an action that was genuinely aimed at protecting consumer and animal health. No scientific study has ever proved an association between the consumption of TSE-affected tissues and the development of CJD. In fact all of the evidence amassed to date implies the opposite.

I managed to pack in a series of lectures during the tour, going down to a nutritional convention near Washington at which I had my speaking time curtailed in favour of someone with more conventional views. I was also given the late night slot, when everyone was exhausted. It was a taxing schedule and I spent ten days lecturing and sleeping on people's couches. The final lecture was sponsored by a Vermont farmer advocacy group called 'Rural Vermont', in the state capital, Montpelier; some important people turned up, including the press. I made a few digs at journalists for not giving fuller and more rigorous coverage to these issues. It's their job to deconstruct the lines they're fed by USDA and others and not accept their statements uncritically. This didn't go down too well with the assembled company.

Over the holiday week I'd spent some time buried in a fascinating book called *The Body Electric*, by Robert Becker and Gary Seldon. Their research work had been carried out at the physics labs at Syracuse University in upstate New York, and it seemed to break new boundaries in the scientific understanding of the electromagnetics of the human body. Over the course of my lecture tour that followed our stay in Vermont I studied this excellent book and followed up its references.

It was at about this time that I had started to think more about the role of the prion protein and Becker had set me thinking in some new directions. I had found most of the attempts at pinning down a role for the prion by the Establishment were lacking in any vision. No one was coming up with any interesting ideas. I was becoming more convinced that being a copper-carrying protein it may have a role in electrical conduction, and when the copper was absent there would be a failure in this function.

Syracuse, nicknamed the 'Salt City', lies in the state of New York, and was named after the original Syracuse in eastern Sicily. It was perhaps coincidence that just as the Greyhound bus pulled into the city I reached a point in Becker's book that produced one of those eureka moments that pulled together many of the missing links in my case book. With the help of his book, I formulated a plausible explanation of my own research findings in the rather oppressive atmosphere of the Greyhound bus station. I was so elated that I felt like proclaiming my breakthrough to the group of rather weary-looking passengers sitting opposite on the hard banquettes of the bus station. I only just restrained myself.

The quantum capacity of metals such as manganese, barium or strontium to absorb light and sound energy can induce a 'Jekyll and Hyde' conversion of these metals from innocuous to toxic forms. I was already aware of the property of certain ferrimagnetic metal compounds based on the trivalent form (3+) of manganese, iron or strontium to absorb the energy of sound. This is well illustrated by the commercial application of these metals in audiotape for storing sound recordings in magnetic form. But I was gripped by the section in Becker's book that highlighted the piezoelectric nature of certain crystals associated with the bone matrix, and their capacity to convert incoming sound or light energy into electrical signals. This association between certain types of crystal and sound energy seemed to suggest a plausible pathogenic mechanism, which would tie my theory up into a unified hypothesis, which accounted for every facet of prion disease. These microcrystals derive from both naturally occurring sources of pollution, such as volcanic emissions, or from industrial sources, such as steel, glass, ceramics, dye manufacture, welding fumes, oil and coal combustion, military explosives, and aerosols to perform radar refraction, nerve gas detection, cloud seeding and rainmaking. The contamination is usually via the nasal-olfactory route, which delivers atmospheric metal microcrystal particulates directly into the brain after inhalation. Once lodged inside the central nervous system, the crystals will bind up with proteins such as the prion and ferritin during periods of copper, sulphur or zinc deficiency and then start to seed the growth of metal-protein crystal arrays in the contaminated tissues. These multireplicated crystals represent the aberrant amyloid fibril and plaque structures, the hallmark of the spongiform diseased brain.

These crystals are piezoelectric in nature and would convert incoming shock bursts of sound and light into electrical signals from sources such as the low-flying jets, military explosions, tectonic shock waves and lightning strikes. The currents would generate magnetic fields, which in turn induce progressive free radical chain reactions of spongiform neurodegeneration.

The TSE brain could be likened to a brain that is contaminated by a million microphone crystals, which will generate deleterious free radical chain reactions immediately the tissues are shock blasted with sound. Once the crucial supply of copper is significantly reduced in the brain, due to deficiency or exposure to copper-chelating chemicals, such as some OP insecticides, then the prion's copper binding sites become vacant, rendering the protein vulnerable to misfolding and bonding with alternative metals. The foreign metal substitution may not act in the best interests of the organism, particularly if the resulting metal seeded crystals are in 'ferrimagnetic' form, i.e. they have the capacity to permanently store up magnetic charge.

Once an individual's brain is contaminated by this form of manganese or barium, any subsequent exposure to external electromagnetic fields such as UV light, sound waves, radar or cell phones will permanently charge up the ferrimagnetically ordered manganese prions. The metals rapidly become permanently saturated with magnetic charge, generating intensive magnetic fields.

So whenever a ferrimagnetically ordered metal is able to substitute at the vacant copper bond on the prion protein, the magnetic field that irradiates from each ferrimagnetically ordered atom will progressively induce contiguous atoms to adopt the same state of ferrimagnetic ordering. This progressively corrupts the circadian and auditory mediated circuits throughout the brain, whereby a state of permanent magnetic charge is spread, domino-style, like a kind of contagious corruption, which jumps across from metal bond to metal bond, from prion to prion. An analogy for this phenomenon is the classic college physics experiment where a magnet is placed alongside a steel nail and the force field of the magnet rapidly magnetizes the adjoining nail.

This theory explains why the so-called 'hyperinfectious' property ascribed to the prion is a misnomer. It is the ferrimagnetic ordering of the metal-seeded prion crystal that serves as the so-called 'infectious' pathogenic agent in TSEs. Whenever TSE research scientists inoculate unfortunate lab animals with TSE brain tissues the rogue crystal components, which carry a magnetic field inducing pathogenic capacity, are passed on into the healthy animal. The crystals rapidly re-seed and multireplicate themselves within the tissues of their new host, and TSE emerges all over again.

The prion protein, albeit misfolded, serves as an innocuous carrier of the crystal 'bullet' into the pathogenic battlefields of the brain. In fact, I think the prion may turn out not to be essential to the disease process at all.

The concept of the ferrimagnetically ordered crystal as the 'TSE agent' also explains why the so-called 'infectious' pathogenic capacity of the TSE agent can survive being heated up to temperatures in excess of 600°C. Ferrimagnetic metals and their crystal structures start to lose their magnetic charge when they are heated above their respective 'Curie point' temperature (e.g., 550°C for manganese 3+).

Barium, silver, manganese and strontium crystals all share the same piezoelectric characteristic — the ability to convert incoming sonic pressure energy into potent pathogenic electrical shocks, which generate a magnetic field around the crystal.

It is interesting that the only way that a vet has to diagnose BSE in a living cow is to apply the simple hand-clap test. If the hand-clap causes the cow to collapse to the ground in writhing agony – as if electric shocks had occurred inside its head – then the vet will give a diagnosis of suspected BSE. This can be likened to the BSE cow having a million piezoelectric microphone crystals lodged inside its brain, which amplify the hand-clap to an unacceptable level. There are also some rather bizarre stories of radio stations being picked up by the mercury crystals inside people's teeth. Well I think much the same is going on in a BSE brain.

These rogue crystal seeds are the primary causal agents in TSEs. They resemble osteoblast generator cells, which are normally involved in the mineralization process of the bone matrix; it's as if these cells have gone astray and been misdirected during embryonic development into the neuronal networks of the brain. Once transplanted, the microcrystals multireplicate themselves during the incubation period, eventually forming substantial metal-protein crystal arrays, such as the fibrils and amyloid plaques, the hallmark of the TSE diseased brain or the helical neurofibrillary tangle features that characterize the neuropathology of the Alzheimer's diseased brain. The brain would appear to become progressively mineralized during these neurodegenerative diseases.

It is interesting that these progenerator cells – the osteoblasts and fibroblasts – are also transmissible. If you transplant these cells from one animal into another, you pass on that ability to be able to generate bone growth in the recipient's tissues – again suggesting that this phenomenon could explain the transmissible facet of the spongiform diseases.

The Nobel Prize-winning scientist Carleton Gajdusek had recorded the presence of substantial deposits of calcium and aluminum in the soft tissues, particularly the neurons, of those who had died of Alzheimer's, ALS and Parkinson's-type neurodegenerative diseases in the South Pacific clusters. Interestingly, Gadjusek had found that these deposits occurred specifically in the form of hydroxyapatites – one of the crystalline materials found in bone. Furthermore, he had found that these abnormal deposits were exclusively located in the areas of the brain that exhibited the pathological damage where the neurofibrillary 'tombstone' tangles occurred, suggesting that these metals could have produced this damage.

The Silicon Valleys

In December 2003 I was contacted by an old friend, Ralph Berney, who used to dairy-farm with his father in the Wensum valley, north-west of Norwich. Ralph pointed out several factors that indicated the valley was an extremely 'hot' location regarding BSE. He felt that whatever was causing this disease was abundantly present in his local environment. Furthermore, Ralph's observations were officially endorsed by the Government's publications that demonstrated excessive rates of BSE in this region of Norfolk throughout the entire duration of the epidemic. He told me that local dairy farms had an embarrassingly high incidence of BSE. Some of the herdsmen who were employed on these farms had been sworn to secrecy over their BSE status in order to maintain the buoyant export trade in top quality replacement pedigree dairy cattle that was practised in the area. In addition one of these herdsmen had sadly died of an early onset Alzheimer-like dementia in his forties. vCJD had also struck in the heart of the local village, where the vicar's wife had sadly died of this grotesque disease. Ralph had been wondering what factors in the valley were causing or promoting the high incidence of TSE. He commented that all of the TSE causal factors that I had raised in my research were very common in the valley: the use of systemic organo-dithiophosphate insecticides for the protection of the local carrot crops against carrot fly; the spreading of copious amounts of manganese and silver contaminated turkey manure across the pastures of the local dairy farms; exposure to frequent daily overflights by low-flying military jets that come from the many military air bases close by. He also felt that the almost unique presence of the battery turkey industry in this area might have played a role, particularly in connection with the liberal use of local turkey manure as a fertilizer on the grassland of all farms that were affected with BSE. He also mentioned the presence of a massive furnace and chimney down by the river that had been used to cook the unwanted waste from the turkey industry, rendering down the remains into a protein feed for live-stock and pet consumption. The acrid odours that used to fumigate the valley had become a hotly contested issue amongst local residents, though the owners of the plant had consistently kept the issue from getting into the local courts.

East Anglia

In September 2004 my brother and I decided to take a trip into the outback of East Anglia to investigate the areas where some of the most intensive clusters of BSE, with the occasional case of vCJD, had erupted in the UK to date.

Our first stop was a World War II airfield at South Pickenham, Norfolk, near where there had been a high incidence of BSE and it was typical of these TSE sites. It is situated just to the north of a major MOD site at Stanford. This area occupies 2227 hectares of the Breckland heath and was first used as an Army training area in 1942 and is still used today for light tank manoeuvres.

When we arrived in the Wensum valley to follow up Ralph Berney's leads, we soon became aware of further connections with World War II. Our investigation took us to a number of murky munition sites, tank shelling ranges and former military air bases, some of which had been redundant since the war. The runways on some of the bases had been taken over in the 1980s and 90s by intensive turkey farms, which had burgeoned in this part of Norfolk but were now for the most part redundant.

The former concrete runways provided an ideal hard standing for the construction of a 'desolation row' of concentration camp style turkey huts, which lay back to back, squatting beneath the wide

Norfolk sky. The retention of the top security military fencing and the search-lamps by the turkey farmers created an eerie atmosphere in these godforsaken locations.

The siting of the huts on the former runways had potentially provided the conditions for the uptake of a cocktail of toxic molecules into the farm food chain. Parts of the runways would carry the persistent residues of metal oxides, which were left behind by the combustion of aircraft fuel and any waste or leaked munitions and, in addition, the toxic legacy of the wartime and cold war accidents that had occurred on these former high security sites. Furthermore, poultry are fed manganese and phosphates to help keep up their growth rates, whilst the silicate-rich fishmeal that was taken from the munition dumping grounds in the North and Irish Seas provided a staple source of protein for the poultry industry during the BSE era.

If you go down to the woods today, you're sure of a big surprise

The first actual cluster of cases of vCJD emerged in one of the most picturesque pockets of the English countryside a few miles west of Ashford in Kent – the so-called Garden of England, a unique pastoral landscape renowned for its swathes of fruit fields, apple orchards and hop farms, with a vibrant agriculture, which is idyllically interwoven between acres of scented flowers and paddocks of grazing sheep. It seemed so incongruous that a disease as grotesque as vCJD should cluster in such beautiful countryside. But lying not far beneath the pastoral façade I rapidly found myself uncovering yet another insidious connection to the UK's World War II chemical munition programme.

I took my first footsteps into the Kentish cluster zone on an early October evening. A sombre mist hung over the wide expanse of the Wealden valley, acting as a kind of reflector for the bleating sheep and a solitary tractor ploughing on a distant farm. A redundant oast-house stood out through the mist like a giant sentry post. I took the footpath through a hop garden and found myself surrounded by a rickety gantry of wires. A few parched bines, still clinging around the strings to the gantry, was all that was left of the rich summer's aisles. There was still a faint antiseptic whiff of hops that hung in the garden and I gathered up a few handfuls of the crisp brown leaves to take home.

The cases of variant and other forms of CJD which were connected to this rural area of Kent (1996–8) added up to a total of ten, although two of the victims were frequent visitors to, rather than full-time residents of, the villages that were implicated.

The vCJD victims included: Susan Carey, whose husband worked on a livestock farm at Mersham, near Ashford; Anna Pearson, a 29-year-old solicitor from Nackington; the first victim of vCJD, Stephen Churchill, who had spent summer holidays at his aunt's dairy farm, which formerly grew hops near Sissinghurst. The family of two other victims of vCJD from Ashford, the sisters Betty Bottle and Joan Stapleden, has long-term connections with Egerton Forstal, the village that appears to represent the centre of this vCJD cluster. Furthermore, father and son, Henry and David Missing, who were originally farmers from Egerton, have both died of the extremely rare type of prion disease known as fatal familial insomnia. This type of CJD is undisputedly caused by an inherited mutation involving the deletion of a select amino acid in the gene that encodes for the prion protein. But what are the factors that seed this mutation in the first instance, enabling this bizarre condition to be passed down from generation to generation?

Other vCJD victims were Graham Brown, a fireman whose family lived at Bethersden village, and Barry Baker, a self-employed woodcutter from the village of High Halden. A further case of vCJD occurred in Clare Tomkins in 1998 who was raised 15 miles to the west in the village of East Peckham, near Tonbridge. In addition to these cases the livestock farms across this whole region had had high rates of BSE, with the second ever recorded outbreak of the disease occurring at Plurendon Manor Farm near Bethersden in early 1985.

Dr Alan Colchester, a consultant neurologist from Guy's Hospital in London, has advanced the only theory to explain this TSE hot-spot. This hypothesis was founded on the official belief that TSEs result from consumption of food products containing TSE-affected tissues. It had blamed the effluent that was discharging into a drainage ditch beside the Canterbury Mills rendering plant at Godmersham — the plant where waste meat by-products were rendered down into this concentrated animal feed.

This drainage ditch was supposed to have contaminated a well that was connected to an aquifer which supplied drinking water to a large area of East Kent. Whilst these allegations had clearly raised important public health issues for the locality, the idea that this pollution had caused the Kentish cluster of CJD was flawed from the start. For only one of the six cases of vCJD that had been linked to Kent was actually in this catchment area for drinking water. So even if the rendering plant had contaminated the drinking water, only one of the victims could have developed the disease as a result.

The TSE villages lie on the western side of Ashford, along an east-west corridor stretching towards Tonbridge, which on first sight seems very similar to the eastern side of Ashford. A casual study of the Ordnance Survey map, however, shows some spatial correlation between the intensive scattering of dewponds and the TSE terri-tories. This could be connected to the fact that these ponds were formed because they had been dug out by previous generations for a source of clay — the geological stratum that underlies this whole region of the Kentish Weald. The surface drainage is therefore poor and tends to retain any toxic pollutants produced in the vicinity on the surface, putting local people at a greater risk of exposure.

Kent has utilized its rich local clay for brick and tile making. Furthermore this clay is particularly rich in silica, and the presence of several brick and pottery works in the area correlates with the consistent presence of the silica risk factor in all other vCJD and sporadic CJD cluster districts in the UK. Interestingly the earliest cases of confirmed BSE had occurred at Pitsham Farm, near Midhurst, which has a specialist brickworks sited at its centre.

During my short stay in these Kentish villages I couldn't help but notice the formidable chimney of the former brickworks at Pluckley, which dominated the landscape, serving as a monument to the enormity of the silicate industry that used to trade in this part of the UK. Set amidst several hundred acres of quarried-out clay pits, the works had closed down about 15 years ago, and the whole site was rapidly reverting to scrubland covered by sapling willows. I was left in little doubt that the area must have been exposed to more than its fair share of silicate particles – piezoelectric microcrystals that could have served to seed the CJD disease process in these local communities.

Silica provides a crucial, fundamental life-giving role and performs as a semiconductor within biological systems. Its role in the body is diverse and contributes to the biological processes of growth, repair, storage of information, organization and rhythmic response. Once those crystals become contaminated by extremely small amounts of impurities, which is deliberately practised in the industrial 'doping' of crystalline materials, then the electrical properties of those crystals are dramatically altered. Once the body is absorbing a steady supply of silicates that have linked with impurities, such as radioactive metals in the external environment, this could be the start of bio-electric problems in the host.

Another intensive source of silicate and other piezoelectric materials is found in munitions and detonators and this turned out to be highly pertinent when I interviewed a local sheep farmer and World War II historian. He and his wife live in Bedlam Lane, which runs in a straight line south-west of the village of Egerton. They kindly set aside their afternoon to show us a collection of fascinating photographs and documentation, which illustrated the activities of the former Canadian and US air force bomber base at

Egerton. The runway, which had been constructed from some commandeered fields opposite his bungalow, had run parallel to Bedlam Lane, passing almost exactly through the point where we were sitting drinking a cup of tea.

I could see a possible explanation for this cluster of CJD. Although no visible sign of the aerodrome remains today, the photos demonstrated that this area of Kent had seen considerable military air force activity during the war. Twelve air bases were concentrated in the area between Egerton and the Kent coast (USAF High Halden being one of them), whilst some of the most advanced bombers of that period, the Thunderbolts, had been flown out of these bases.

Hand in hand with the intensive presence of the military went the intensive exposure of the local environment to megatons of munitions. These were dispensed by the militaries on both sides of the World War II conflict. Indeed the cluster area lay directly beneath the infamous air route known as 'Bomb Alley' – the well-worn flight path used by German bombers, which operated daily sorties between Germany and the UK. The CJD cluster area lay beneath the point at which the German bombers were forced to dump their bomb load, due to fears of last minute fuel shortages or the need to escape the British fighter planes in hot pursuit. The German propelled missiles known as Doodlebugs had also been directed towards the heart of London along the same Bomb Alley route. According to the *Kent Messenger* newspaper, 2400 Doodlebugs had fallen short of their London target and exploded in the Kent countryside, showering the environment in metal microcrystals. Our host had charted the exact locations in Egerton and Smarden where hundreds of these displaced incendiary and high explosive bombs had been dropped. He also described the frequency of plane crashes and munition accidents; they were an almost daily occurrence at the air base. One photo of a Flying Fortress bomber that had crashed into a Kentish oast house at Southenden Farm bore full witness to his statement.

A lead from the internet had taken me into the nearby Frith, Dering and Foxden Woods in search of the remnants of World War II bomb stores. I focused on the most important central thread of this investigation – the UK's World War II chemical weapons programme of chemical ordnance production. Dering Wood served as an encampment for troops who were waiting for orders to be dispatched to the D-Day landings. The northern end of the woodland, known as Frith Woods, was used for bomb and ammunition storage. Another dump for World War II munitions had been an old quarry adjoining the former windmill on Stonehill. But I became particularly interested in another woodland that surrounded Egerton House, known as Foxden Woods. It had been referred to as the 'ammo dump' by the local community, who remembered a tightly guarded system of security in place during the war years – one that was considerably more intense than the other seemingly similar bomb stores in the area. In fact, the whole area was cordoned off by the military. This wood seemed especially relevant, because all of the relatives of the CJD victims who I'd been able to track down and engage in discussion with had reported that the victims had regularly played in these woods as children. It seems that they had also eaten significant amounts of blackberries, hazelnuts, fungi and wild game such as rabbit, pheasant and pigeon from this woodland. In fact, a pheasant shooting syndicate has been operating in these woods up to the present day.

David Missing, the Egerton farmer's son, who like his father had actually died of the inherited type of CJD disease fatal familial insomnia, had taken a keen interest in the military history of the local woodlands. He collected various supposedly innocuous memorabilia, such as shells and bombs that he had found in the woods over the years. His widow still has them in the family home today. It appears that Foxden Woods had served as one of the main chemical bomb depots during World War II and the munitions had been stockpiled in readiness for supplying the local bomber base at Egerton.

Although I have no conclusive evidence for this, it is documented that Churchill had located these chemical armouries in woodlands adjoining airfields all the way down the eastern side of the UK, from Lossiemouth to Kent, in readiness for a last ditch attempt to repel a German invasion. The intensive military presence surrounding Foxden Woods suggested that storage had occurred here. The local people also mentioned a rather bizarre 'over the top' response from the authorities after a local farmer had recently reported discovering what was thought to be a rather ordinary relic of a World War II incendiary bomb in a nearby dewpond. Specialist bomb disposal squads were called from all over the UK to deal with this supposedly 'ordinary' find!

I gathered up my sampling gear and turned off the road into what appeared to be the former entrance into the old bomb dump. The bough of a decrepit looking oak tree had slumped across the entrance of the track, making access difficult. A curtain of ivy hung from the main trunk, darkening the undergrowth of the gloomy woodland still further. I kept my head down and pushed through some thickets; a flicker of light broke through the treetops above, adding a little warmth to this sinister place. It was silent and the total lack of birdsong made me anxious. A little further into the woodland and I found an old pad of concrete under a cover of autumn leaves and assumed that this was the base pad for some kind of sentry post. A little deeper still and I found an extensive area of ground where several pits had been dug. A fine coating of moss had covered everything, lending a lunar-like quality to the scene.

I dug some samples from the old pits, sensing that these might be the 'ammo dump' referred to by the local people. Quite rapidly, I seemed to be overcome by an instant feeling of nausea and fatigue, accompanied by an acute sore throat and dizziness. I wondered about the rabbits, which had burrowed down to make their homes in these pits. An analysis of their tissues would provide a more reliable scientific indicator for gauging the presence of a nerve agent than my own reaction to the site.

The other possible source of munition fallout in this area of Kent could be the substantial military firing ranges located along the coastline at Lydd and Hythe, about 15 miles south of the CJD region. The Lydd range is actually famous for its development of picric acid or lyddite as it became known. This piezoelectric munition material was used as a detonator for military explosives, and many thousands of tons of this and other classes of munition have been tested on these ranges over the years. Since the metal microcrystals that result from the physical forces of the explosion become airborne, it is feasible that these micro-particles are usually blown inland from the testing ranges by the sea, and their fallout is subsequently deposited in a bandwidth along the entire length of the Wealden valley. The advent of testing with the new generation of depleted uranium munitions during the 1980s could have con-siderably exacerbated the problem of exposure to microcrystals in the Kentish cluster region.

Incidence of scrapie in the flocks of Romney sheep that have traditionally grazed the marshes around the Lydd and Hythe ranges is known to be high. In this particular type of scrapie, a mutation in the prion protein gene has been shown to underpin the disease. Once again, it seems that high-dose exposure of mammals to these types of munition contamination will cause a mutation in the region of the gene (usually in the sulphur-rich residues), which the pol-lutant tends to target and form a stable bond with during embryonic development. Lower exposure may induce the 'sporadic' forms of TSE, where no mutation has been identified.

Local sheep farmers such as Gary Coomber from Headcorn have reported abnormal neurological disturbances in sheep that have grazed down on the marshes around the military ranges. Once again, the toxic characteristics of the CJD cluster environment in Kent appear to fulfil all of the prerequisites of my theory. For example, the atmospheric drifting of systemic organophosphates and 245T in the intensive strawberry, broad bean and apple crop-ping that is so characteristic of this region of Kent would have most probably compromised the function of the blood-brain barriers of the exposed population. This may enable an increased uptake and 'leakage' of microcrystals across this normally effective barrier and into the brain.

The cultivation of hops in the UK is virtually exclusive to this area of Kent, and the Ministry of Agriculture's pesticide usage surveys have shown that hops tend to be treated with a hundred higher levels of organophosphate pesticides than the commonly cultivated cereal crops. A major accident at ICI Zeneca's pesticide plant at Yalding in Kent (15 miles to the west) on 17 April 1986 involving the release of gas from a tanker containing a precursor chemical for an organophosphate pesticide could have further exacerbated OP exposure amongst residents of the valley. One of the victims of vCJD, 24-year-old Clare Tomkins, was raised in the village of East Peckham, which is little more than one mile across the meadows from the Yalding pesticide factory. She had been a committed vegetarian for eleven years prior to the onset of her CJD symptoms.

The sonic shock perspective of the Kent CJD is as evident as in the other locations and this provides a temporal explanation for the cluster. Local people report that immediately prior to the Gulf War there was constant low flying by Tornado jets travelling in an east-west direction across the middle of the cluster area, following the route of the main-line railway to London. The local people at Headcorn told me that they had endured more than their fair share of jet overflights and they had ascribed this to the fact that the trainer pilot in charge of the squadron was dating a girl who lived in the Smarden vicinity. The pilot was deliberately passing over the vicinity to show off his skills to his fiancé! Local children also report being terrified by the overflights, complaining of the complete lack of warning of the approaching planes. The local people seemed relieved that there had been a substantial reduction in these over-flights over the last five years.

My working hypothesis suggests that these sonic shocks activate and promote the 'dormant' piezoelectric microcrystals that have been deposited in the brains of the exposed local population. During incubation the crystals multireplicate into the full-fledged rogue fibril structures that are the hallmark of the neuropathology of the TSE diseased brain, thereby unleashing their latent pathogenic capacity. The acoustic pressure waves are converted into electric shocks, which invoke the cascade of free radical mediated neurodegeneration, which results in the spongiform holes in the brain. The actual timing of the main burst of these sonic challenges was from 1990 to 2000 in Kent and correlates with the period of outbreak of these vCJD cases from 1995 to 1998. Other sources of sonic challenge in the area link to the incoming and outgoing flights of aircraft from Headcorn Airport, as well as the constant passage of overflights entering London's Heathrow Airport.

All of the environments surrounding the other 'mini-clusters' of vCJD in the UK fit this pattern of dual exposure to silicaceous microcrystals as a primary prerequisite and sonic shock bursts as a secondary prerequisite. For example, eleven cases of vCJD emerged in the Strathclyde region around Glasgow, in the small settlements of Motherwell, Coatbridge, Harthill, Eaglesham, Yoker, Milton of Campsie, Moodiesburn, Bearsden and Erskine. The presence of a large munition factory at Bishopton combined with the frequent overflights of aeroplanes using Glasgow Airport pinpoints the local sources of the causal prerequisites in this particular cluster of vCJD.

Whilst the Bishopton plant was 'the largest ordnance factory ever erected in the UK, producing the country's principal source of cordite, TNT and RDX explosives during the Second World War', it was operated as a Royal Ordnance factory right up until the time that it was decommissioned in 2002. The issue of disposal of the thousands of tons of waste ordnance has recently posed a major environmental hurdle for the local community. It has been reported that a substantial tonnage of this waste has been incinerated in the locality, showering the local communities with these microcrystal pollutants. Once again, this distribution of cases around but not in the main conurbation area begs the question: if tainted beef consumption were the cause, why have all of the cases of vCJD erupted in the small rural satellite settlements? Surely you would expect the majority of cases to be in the main conurbation area of highest population density?

This must indicate that some phenomenon confined to rural areas underlies the cause of these outbreaks of vCJD. Given that airports and their flight paths plus facilities linked to munition manufacture and testing are invariably sited away from areas of high population density, then the persistent presence of these phenomena within TSE cluster areas could offer a plausible explanation for this curious rural pattern.

Maple Leaf Rage

The New Year came in with a flurry of light snow which settled over our hill farm. It covered the rutted tracks and cast a soft white shroud on the back of 2004. The purity of that morning was tainted by a series of desperately sad emails from a group of Canadian family ranchers. Two fresh cases of mad cow disease had been diagnosed in Alberta, and had clearly thrown the rural communities into a state of despair. Following on from a year of US border closure, which had virtually ruined the country's cattle sales, combined with a pile-up of cows without sufficient feed, this news has penetrated deep into the heart of Canadian rural culture, driving a hard-working community closer to the brink of extinction.

In health risk terms, these two new cases of BSE do not warrant alarm since it seems to me to be little different from a couple of cows walking around with a neurodegenerative disease, i.e. I do not believe it is contagious. In respect of the total number of BSE cases that Canada has experienced – a mere three cases to date – it's completely insignificant. Great Britain has suffered 250,000 plus cases of BSE, which makes one wonder why there has been such a vehement degree of scaremongering over three BSE cows in a country as large as Canada.

My tiny farm in the UK has suffered three cases of BSE, yet thankfully we never had to endure invasion by a slaughter squad or be zipped up in space suits or have the farm closed as a biohazard zone. BSE for us arrived with some bought-in pedigree cattle, yet it never spread to our own home-reared animals despite twelve months of intermingling between the two groups. Our own BSE problem went away with the affected animals in the slaughter wagon, and has never appeared again. This same 'non-infectious' pattern of BSE was exhibited by all of the 250,000 BSE cases that struck the British Isles. Since we have the benefits of a long epidemiological history on BSE behind us now, why do the global health authorities choose to panic. In health risk terms, do these Canadian BSE cases actually warrant the virtual shutting down of the entire family farming community of Canada? I think not.

The question that the US Department of Agriculture (USDA) and the Canadian Government need to be asking is: how did these two cows develop BSE if they never ate tainted meat and bone meal feed, the supposed cause of BSE? Unfortunately, the UK Government could never face up to this most obvious and pressing question — which is strange, since over 43,000 cows that were born after the 1988 ban on this feed in the UK have still gone down with BSE. Further cases have occurred after the second 'reinforced' ban of 1996. Furthermore, many European countries have now had more cases of BSE in cows born after their respective bans than in cows born before their bans. Canada has now joined this ever-growing list.

One of the most important US cattle groups, known as R-Calf, were not helping matters. In fact, their actions to sue the USDA for rightly planning to lift the block on Canadian beef imports across the border was misguided. R-Calf's actions were ultimately shooting their ranching businesses in the foot. They were merely feeding the myth of the mad cow 'crisis', which will devour them all in the end.

R-Calf was trying to blockade Canadian beef imports on the basis of an unproven argument — that the hyperinfectious protein-only contagion contained in BSE-affected beef poses a grave threat to US livestock and human health.

When I lectured to a group of farmers at Billings in Montana, one of the contributors from the floor raised the issue of a live cow and infected feed study conducted in the UK. He thought this work provided the ultimate evidence in support of the current hyper-infectious paranoia of the global health authorities. This single experiment involved the successful induction of BSE in 11 of 16 cows that had been fed varying oral doses (1 g, 10 g, 100 g, 300 g) of brainstem homogenate taken from BSE-affected cows.

Firstly, in the real world cattle don't eat homogenate at all, let alone in a concentrated form like this. They ate MBM feed, a tiny fraction of which may have contained BSE prions. More to the point, they don't even eat MBM now as it has been banned for years. The BSE material would have been vastly 'diluted' by the mass of bulking nutriment used in feed manufacture. Therefore the experiment didn't replicate either the dosage that an 'on-farm' cow would be likely to consume or the exact form and context of the dose. Furthermore, this does not mean that animals living together in their normal way would then pass on BSE through bodily fluids for example.

But even if transmission was successful in these trials, with some animals developing clinical BSE, we must remember that transmission does not necessarily imply an infection. You could be transmitting a toxic, heat-resistant metal-protein microcrystal from the diseased animal, that re-seeds itself once it is implanted into the brain of a new host.

But the UK Government's account of this study seems to vary dramatically — depending on whom is being told about it. The fact that these trial cows had been purchased off an ordinary British farm from which they might have contracted BSE (and remember, BSE is probably seeded in early life, perhaps even during 'in utero' stages) indicates that these studies were scientifically flawed from the outset. And the small number of cows involved also invalidates the usefulness of the trial — whatever the outcome.

The fact that the whole world has designed its BSE policy on the back of such a small study is curious, to say the least. Whenever governments have called their opposing forces to provide evidence at public inquiries (such as myself), they rightly deem it imperative that any evidence submitted to the hearings must be substantial and have already been profiled in the peer-reviewed academic literature.

But, true to form, it is one set of rules for the Establishment and another, far more stringent set for their opponents.

Furthermore, the UK Government has been giving out contra-dictory statements on both the protocols and timing/dates of this study. For some of my Canadian rancher friends, the Czar family, had written to the UK Government asking about these tests and were told in the response that this experiment was still in progress (and only a total of 'ten cows' involved) and would be published shortly. But, seven years ago, a very reliable MAFF official and a vet, Mr Tom Eddy, had informed my brother Nigel of these live cow tests and how they already had been completed with positive results. Again, I can't find a peer-reviewed publication that describes the research. Nine months ago, the Government informed me that these trials were complete and the results had been sub-mitted to the EU Commission. But in the absence of any journal publication, what are we to believe?

Unfortunately, I have to say that the UK Government exhibits a track record of disseminating misinformation into the public domain – and North America has become their latest victim in the propaganda campaign over the true cause of BSE. For the UK Government has an awful lot to hide in order to dodge a liability issue here.

North American government officials would do well to question the validity of the statements in the Gabriel Horne Report on the origins of BSE. This report has been spun across the breadth of America and Canada and is hailed as a flagship publication, which charters the gospel according to the UK Government on all issues surrounding BSE. But in truth this document uses disinformation and misrepresentation whilst making a judicial selection of the data in order to funnel the outside world into the UK Government's agenda on BSE. Despite being authored by several leading pro-fessors, the report does not stand up to scrutiny.

In order to persuade the US and Canadian Governments to dis-card my research data, the UK Government has promoted the

Horne Report, which misleads the reader over many issues. For example, according to Horne the OP warble fly treatment ceased in 1982. According to the UK Diseases of Animals Act and 'The Warble Fly Order England and Wales 1982' it started in 1982. The report states: 'since the majority of cows which developed BSE were born after 1982 [true], and the use of organophosphates for warble control had ceased by 1982 [false], then how can BSE be associated with exposure to these organophosphate warble fly compounds.' I find it hard to believe (or do I?) that the British Department of Agriculture cannot remember the start date of the Act, which they themselves had formulated for the UK Parliamentary Statute Book. Ironically, I was in court in 1985 to challenge the same Act in order to prevent compulsory treatment of my own cattle! There are many other flaws in the report, which I have dealt with in more detail in my chapter on BSE.

The UK Government is obviously worried about the threats of any potential liabilities that might arise from any further validation of my work – particularly if a primary role of an organophosphate in the pathogenesis of BSE is proven. Thus, in accord with my theory, it was the Government's compulsory treatment of bovines with these systemic acting organophosphate nucleating agents, used at exclusively high dose rates in the UK, that is a major factor in the cause of this disease. The OP oil-based formulation was poured along the spine of the cow, millimetres from the central nerves where the BSE disease process is first initiated. The OP fulfilled a number of functions, which I would link with BSE pathogenesis, such as chelation of copper and sulphur and up-regulating the host's manufacture of prion protein.

These rogue crystals are piezoelectric by nature, and therefore compromise the ability of the contaminated individual to deal with intense sound waves in the normal manner. This disrupts the homeostasis of electrochemical signalling in the brain, and sets off a chain reaction of free radical mediated spongiform neuro-degeneration in the cow's brain.

The strange thing about the current situation in the Canadian cattle battle is that nobody in authority seems to care about the plight of their own rural community, which is particularly ironic because these communities provide a key role in propping up the Canadian economy. The few who actually get CJD are just told that the disease has no cure, and are sent home to die. Stranger still, is the total betrayal by the Canadian Government (or any government for that matter) of the best interests of its own people. There seems to be a deep-rooted inertia that afflicts decision makers, whereby the status quo is clung to because it does not involve risk in decision making or thoroughness in research. BSE has been drummed up into a major political, cultural and economic threat, when all along the science behind the story indicates that this disease is not a simple infection but a complex, multifactorial disease.

Whilst we clearly need to investigate and eradicate the disease we can only begin to achieve this by identifying and accepting the disease's true cause. The official inertia that has been adopted by the Canadian Establishment towards its ailing rural communities is transformed into enthusiastic cooperation when it comes to new ventures with the multinationals. Yet I believe the multinationals are forging a lucrative business out of BSE. They need people to be scared of BSE, in order that they can market multi-million pound packages of 'live cow BSE tests', BSE-resistant GM cows, or – better still – replace the world's 'dangerously infected' meat and milk protein supply with their own genetically modified package of chemically grown, sterile GM arable protein crops.

The Canadian mandarins are feeding the very multinational monster that is draining the blood from their own people. The multinational policy for global takeover of the protein supply is being exercised by a handful of key individuals from the corporate world who have installed themselves into prime positions of power in virtually every country. In Canada, their field officers have worked their way into the upper echelons of the Canadian agri-world – the deer and cattle associations – where they are representing anything but the best interests of their own membership. It's much the same here in the UK, where the corporations have installed their own representatives into the UK Government's Civil Service. They operate on the principle that if you place your people on both sides of the chessboard then you will be sure to win the game.

It is not a game, though, for the ranchers, because their culture represents generations of hard work, intuitive wisdom and a lifestyle that requires an immense degree of inner integrity to sustain. And so we prepare to sit back and watch a chunk of our agricultural heritage going down the pan, to appease the short-term profits of a handful of global tycoons – all for the purchase of products for which we have little need. The root of the problem seems to stem from the fact that too many vested interests have become involved in the business of BSE. The government departments are simply not interested in anything that challenges the commercial master plan.

A number of 'Bio' companies are working up their marketplace in Canada right now. Most of these internationally based companies are connected back to one of the leading global corporations, who have been only too keen to keep the main governments hypnotized by the hyperinfectious 'health risks' posed by BSE. This is aimed at coercing governments to give the 'nod' to the mass marketing of their four dollar per cow live BSE test, so that it cajoles every single rancher across North America into buying their test – not to mention their scheme to unleash GM prion protein knock out cows (guaranteed BSE resistant) onto the farm scene.

This indicates that there is a great deal of money at stake for these companies. But what they have overlooked is the overall effect of their sustained campaign of scaremongering and its negative repercussions on the economic status of the farming community at large. The critical swathe of media words against livestock farmers over recent years has been sufficient to impoverish our farmlands.

It is therefore hard to see how the multinationals will be able to market their four dollar per cow BSE live test, since the impact of their propaganda to get governments to run with their tests has ironically ended up rendering the poor old cow totally worthless.

One way forward is to plead with our governments that they return to the days when they acted more independently of commercial interests. We need them to call into question all of the junk science that has been laid down about the origins of BSE, and get them to reopen a truly independent investigation into the origins of this complex disease.

Behind the Iron Curtain

European livestock farmers dread the day when their cattle succumb to a tuberculosis breakdown. The implications are severe: a ruthless cull of infected cattle and badgers, with all remaining healthy cattle impounded behind a curtain of government mandated movement restrictions and red tape. The effect has been to propel small farming businesses into a state of financial meltdown. But the official procedures of TB control are archaic and outmoded. They are founded on the old hypothesis that humans develop TB as a sole result of exposure to TB-infected animals, and at the same time failing to accommodate the more recent discoveries in the multifactorial science surrounding mycobacterial disease. We need to be questioning whether such cruel and costly strategies currently involved in TB control programmes are actually achieving their desired effect – to protect the human population against the TB agent.

In the summer of 2005 I was forced to come to terms with my own cattle joining the ever-increasing ranks of TB-infected herds which are currently blighting the UK.

At dawn I scaled the hill to collect the cattle from my outlying fields. The earth still retained some of the heat of the previous day, and I was forced to goad the cows because they seemed more reluctant than usual to rise and amble to the nearby lane. Perhaps they were more perceptive than I was, sensing the fate that was approaching.

As we reached the steep gradient of the shillet track, the cattle accelerated a little, rutting up the dust with their hooves. The swish of a cow's tail disturbed an early morning bee that droned off beyond the bank of bluebells and into the haze of the dazzling sun.

Gradually the entire caravan of cattle wended its way down the track to the bottom of the valley. On the last stretch to the farm, a patch of giant foxgloves towered over us, displaying their luminescent red and mauve lanterns. But I failed to heed the red alert, and just drove the cows on without a second thought.

Back at the yard, the vet was ready and we led the cows straight down to the inspection pens. The procedure was simple – to measure the size of any lumps that had erupted on the cows' necks. This serves as a yardstick for gauging the extent of the allergic response to the TB skin test – an intradermal injection of tubercle bacillus that had been administered by the vet three days earlier. After a few minutes I saw the vet stand back abruptly. 'Oh,' he said in a despondent, drawn out tone, popping on his spectacles slightly askew, 'we could have a problem here, Mark.' I watched him fumbling through his pockets for the callipers, and now knew that he had to take a more precise measurement of what obviously looked like a colossal reaction lump on the cow's neck. I became anxious, and my mouth was becoming parched in anticipation of what was coming next. The air was heavy, like the lull before a thunderstorm. Even the robins, who had been busy in the yard a minute earlier rustling up the brittle leaves, had become silent. The vet raised his glasses and wiped the sweat off his forehead. 'You have a reactor, I'm afraid, Mark.'

A few minutes later there was another reactor, and then several more. My mouth had become more parched and my stomach felt nauseous. I became angry at the thought of these fine young pedigree animals, just into their prime, condemned to slaughter under the Government's animal health diktat.

Like many other cattle farmers in the UK, I was confused by the perfect condition of the TB-reactor cows, since I had always assumed that TB was a debilitating disease. Although these cows had reacted to the skin test and were therefore deemed to carry TB, I began to wonder whether they had successfully adapted to the infection by knocking out the greater majority of the invasive mycobacteria. The TB slaughter programme could actually be annihilating the resistant animals – culling the genetically robust individuals that we really needed to be keeping as breeding stock for future generations.

The next stage of the so-called 'crisis' procedure was to retire to the farmhouse to fill out a tree's worth of forms and several sheets of a TB questionnaire. I was amazed by the simplistic contents of the questions. Each one was based on the assumption that the transmission of the TB agent from infected badgers to cattle was the sole cause of bovine TB. *Baddie the badger* had been dubbed the culprit before the necessary detective work had even begun. The same 'back-to-front' investigation was applicable to the questionnaire which the Government presented to farms that had experienced a case of mad cow disease. The whole thing was very simplistic and every question was based on the assumption that the cause was meat and bone meal, despite evidence which indicated that this theory was flawed. The same was true of the variant CJD questionnaire.

The real question for me was why had my farm always boasted a TB-free status, despite being surrounded by TB-affected cattle and badgers for many years. I began to wonder what changes had been integrated into my farming practices over recent years – changes that could be responsible for switching on the susceptibility of our cattle to the TB agent. I felt that this was the essential question to be answered.

TB is virtually endemic in the soils, waters and atmospheres of the majority of ecosystems, where mycobacteria have co-existed with mammalian life for centuries. Despite its widespread prevalence, the TB agent has produced relatively few major outbreaks across the world. It seems that an epidemic of clinical TB can only erupt once some anti-TB component of our immune defence has been disrupted. In this respect, the primary event is a disruption of immunity, which enables the TB agent to breach the body's defences and opportunistically take a hold.

A historical study of the epidemiology of TB demonstrates that epidemics of TB have occurred since the Iron Age, and that this disease has always been rife amongst specific population groups who are nutritionally impoverished in some way. For example, TB was rife amongst city slum dwellers, who had no choice but to breath the industrially polluted air 24 hours a day, as well as the half-starved Scottish and Irish crofters who were evicted during the clearances and forced onto boats bound for North America. Another more recent example involves AIDS victims whose immune systems are so severely compromised that they invariably develop TB as a secondary complication.

What is the key factor that has suddenly unleashed TB susceptibility amongst my cattle following so many years of TB-free status? After much thought about the recent specific changes that I had integrated into my farming system, I began to wonder whether the TB breakdown in my herd could be connected to the drastic cost-cutting measures which I have been forced to adopt in order to survive in farming.

Along with most other livestock farmers across the UK, we had foolishly cut back on the use of the so-called 'non-essential' lime and calcified seaweed based fertilizers. The trend in reduced usage of lime based fertilizers has been exacerbated by recent conservation measures that have debarred the harvesting of Cornish calcified seaweed altogether, thereby preventing future usage of this material on the farm.

The general reduction in use of lime fertilizers, combined with the recent increases in winter rainfall across the western UK, has acidified the topsoil as a result. Other influences such as acid rain and the continued use of so called 'essential' artificial fertilizers will be playing a role in the acidification of agricultural ecosystems.

The pH of the soil on our farm has dropped from an acceptably neutral 6 to an acidic 5 over the last three years. This is backed up by the invasion of buttercups into our pastures where clover used to flourish.

Research has shown that there is a correlation between areas of high mycobacteria incidence and regions where the soils are acidic. This association is strengthened by the results of studies in which lime was spread on farms in Michigan that were suffering from high rates of mycobacterium infection (albeit the paratuberculosis strain of mycobacterium). The study concluded that the lime treatment had produced a tenfold reduction in the infection of cattle after a three-year period had passed.

The relevant issue in respect of TB infection and soil acidity hinges on the fact that acidification of the topsoil leads to an excessive accumulation of available iron, particularly in the regions where soil iron is naturally elevated and rainfall is high. The iron is taken up by the pasture herbage, especially ryegrass and plantain, and bluebell bulbs and also percolates into the local water supplies as a result. Animals then eat and drink of these high iron resources.

Interestingly, the key hotspot zones of bovine TB across the UK are the Forest of Dean, Exmoor, Cornwall, Devon and the Mendip Hills. These regions all correlate with the areas where iron has been mined in abundance and rainfall is high. Preliminary pasture sampling from the specific fields on my own farm (June 2005) where the TB-reactors had been pastured has consistently demonstrated an excessive elevation of iron (average 378 mg/kg) in relation to the levels of 143 mg/kg recorded three years previously. This research is being expanded to cover TB-free and TB farms across the key TB cluster areas of the UK.

Much research published in the scientific literature indicates that iron represents an essential prerequisite in the pathogenesis of TB, enabling TB and other strains of mycobacterium to proliferate, metabolize and survive within the mammalian biosystem. It is the supply of 'free' iron within the host that provides the TB agent with its enhanced capacity to unleash its pathogenicity.

Although TB victims adapt to their parasitic attacks by storing their iron supplies in tissues that are inaccessible to the mycobacteria, the disease process culminates in the parasite getting the upper hand with the host developing the classic iron-deficient anaemic state that is a central clinical feature of TB.

Mycobacteria acquire their iron from the host's own transferrin and ferritin molecules – the iron binding transport and storage proteins that are integral to the healthy metabolism of iron within the mammals. The mycobacteria take iron from their host by releasing a type of iron-capturing siderophore called an exochelin, which in turn transfers and donates the iron back to the mycobactins which exist in the cell walls of the mycobacteria themselves.

This hijaking of the host's iron supply is beneficial for the survival of the TB mycobacteria in more ways than one. Not only does the TB agent utilize the host's iron for its own proliferation and survival, but it also utilizes this metal to indemnify its own long-term security within the host by disabling the host's immune defence against itself. The parasite achieves this means of self–protection by preventing the viable synthesis of the iron-binding beta-2-microglobulin molecules whose role is to activate the killer T-lymphocytes – the host's main line of defence against mycobacterial infection. This could explain why humans whose T-cell immune defence has become compromised through nutritional deprivation, chemical exposure or AIDS are at a significantly greater risk of developing TB as a secondary complication.

TB is not the only pathogen that depends upon the host's iron for its maintenance and growth within the body. *Clostridium botulinum* (implicated in grass sickness of horses), leprosy, HIV, *Candida*, *Listeria*, *Salmonella* and malaria are all members of this insidious family of ironmonger pathogens to which TB belongs.

Only last week, champion horsebreeder Gail Dunsbee contacted me about the sudden death of one of her horses as a result of grass sickness – a devastating paralysis of the autonomic nerve endings in the horse's gut due to infection with *Clostridium botulinum*. But much like TB, *C. botulinum* is virtually endemic in the alimentary tract of horses where it rarely produces any adverse health effects at all. So what environmental factor had suddenly enabled the infection to flourish?

Dissatisfied with the professional ignorance surrounding the causes of grass sickness, Gail had taken matters into her own hands in order to safeguard the future of her surviving horses. And it looks as if the results of her preliminary soil analyses have provided the causal clues to this catastrophic problem for horse breeders.

Apart from the low potassium readings, the excessively high readings for iron (at 1344 ppm) comprised the only other element of the twelve elements tested which had deviated from its respective reference range. This result could explain why grass sickness, like TB, has invariably remained confined to acid soil districts where iron levels are generally elevated.

Since elevated iron increases TB risk, it is easy to understand how the management of dietary iron can influence the outcome of TB. For example, when TB-infected mice were treated with the iron-chelating lactoferrin protein (a natural ingredient of colostrum milk), there was a hundredfold reduction in the number of pathogens present in the mice.

Likewise, individuals suffering from TB used to be regularly treated with the iron-chelating compound p-aminosalicylate with some success. It could prove beneficial from a preventative as well as a curative perspective to introduce copper or zinc bicarbonate supplements into the diet of TB-affected populations. Whilst these anionic compounds do not act as iron chelators as such, they will impair the absorption of iron across the alimentary tract by competing for its uptake system of transport proteins. Any foodstuffs containing phytic acids, such as alfalfa, clover and grains, will also produce the same anti-iron effects.

The use of inorganic phosphorus as an inclusion in fertilizers or mineral feed supplements would also assist in reducing the amount of free iron that is rendered 'available' in the soil or taken up into the animal respectively. The phosphorus competes for the iron-binding site on the transport proteins that normally convey iron across the gut wall, thereby arresting the uptake of iron at its initial point of entry into the body.

It is also important to consider the knockout effects that iron chelators might have upon the other pathogens that need to bite the iron bullet before they can trigger disease. For instance, it has already been demonstrated that the iron-chelating compounds deferoxamine and 8-hydroxyquinoline-5-sulphonic acid have produced beneficial effects in the treatment of leprosy and *Clostridium botulinum* respectively.

My proposal is that badgers and cattle that co-exist within the same environments will both develop TB due to their separate co-exposure to the same iron-rich food chain, and not necessarily due to a cross-infection from one animal to the other. Bluebell and other iron-rich bulbs/roots constitute a large part of the badger's diet and these will gradually load up the badger's biosystem with iron until threshold levels are exceeded, thereby providing any mycobacterial pathogens that are present with the sustenance to proliferate to pathogenic levels. Likewise, the high incidence of human TB that has been recorded amongst steelworkers and slum dwellers who lived beside their workplaces during the industrial revolution could have been induced by the high levels of iron in the atmospheres of their local environment.

I believe that government ministers in the UK have been correct in resisting pressures to re-enact wholesale slaughter of badgers as a means of controlling TB in the bovine and human populations. For the badger culls in previous years have achieved nothing in terms of eradicating TB. The disease has kept on recurring irrespective of the various slaughter measures that have been put in place. We need to consider what is actually achieved each time that we re-enact this drastic, unnecessary solution of badger gassing and blanket cattle culls for TB control.

Furthermore, it is scientifically naive to think that we will ever be able to eradicate a pathogen that is endemic in the environment at large. As long as optimum eco-conditions for the survival of TB mycobacterium are allowed to exist, such as high iron and soil acidity, then TB epidemics will continue to occur as and when alterations in weather conditions and husbandry methods permit.

In respect of consumers who are anxious about exposure to TB pathogens in their foods, they need to be aware that modern methods of food processing safeguard consumers from exposure to the TB agent – methods which didn't exist half a century ago. For example, any milk that is taken from a TB-affected animal today is automatically pasteurized in the modern dairy set-up. Although pasteurization produces some negative health effects, by switching our immune response to TB and other pathogens into 'sleep mode', this ultra-efficient sterilization process provides a guarantee for those who are concerned about TB exposure.

The type of practical control measures that I advocate are low tech and inexpensive. Unfortunately there seems to be a deep-rooted antipathy towards non-trendy low-tech solutions in our society and this usually works against such ideas being taken up. Whilst it is high time that governments should say farewell to their archaic strategy for TB control, some viable alternative will be needed to replace it. Governments should begin to examine the considerably cheaper, animal welfare friendly option of encouraging farmers (via subsidies) to adopt husbandry practices that prevent cattle from succumbing to TB infection in the first instance. This could be achieved through subsidizing the spreading of lime fertilizers across the TB-endemic regions, as well as promoting feeding and fertilizing with iron-chelating or anti-iron compounds on farms in the TB risk areas. This would reduce the amount of iron flowing up the farm food chain, which in turn would reduce the levels of TB mycobacteria.

Such a radical approach, which reduces the susceptibility of cattle to the TB agent, could produce some major advantages over the existing system which simply slaughters infected animals. This would achieve a considerable reduction in the overall incidence of

TB, thereby reaping major savings for both human and animal life, farmers' livelihoods and the taxpayer.

Since the incidence of TB is increasing amongst the human population, it is high time that we adopted a more intelligent, civilized and updated strategy for dealing with the prevention of TB. We should be taking a closer look at the underlying causes of 'iron overload' in the human food chain and ecosystem at large. This would entail looking at the impact of acid rain and how it brings about a rise in the levels of available iron within the soil and water supplies. Issues surrounding the industrial emission of iron parti-culates into the atmosphere, as well as the supplementation of our foods with iron additives represent important areas that warrant investigation and the development of controls.

Likewise, the indirect impact of various toxic or mutagenic environmental agents upon the metabolic processes that regulate iron homeostasis is an area that also needs to be considered. Many environmental chemicals and metals are recognized to disrupt the body's capacity to regulate the balanced uptake, storage and/or excretion of iron, thereby representing an alternative means through which iron levels could become elevated in the biosystem, which in turn leads to an increased susceptibility to TB infection.

*

Meanwhile, back on my farm as night fell, the knacker man arrived to collect my TB-reactor cows. I lead the unsuspecting cows to the loading pen, feeling guilty that I had betrayed them by failing to mount any kind of resistance against the Government's strategy of senseless slaughter. The cows waited in the half-light with their backs steaming and their heads held low as they savoured their final moments of freedom.

The death wagon rattled down my long farm track and then backed up to the loading pen. The ramps came down and after a chorus of whelping and lashing of hooves, the cows slid and clat-tered up the steel ramp into the dark belly of the lorry. The tailgate was securely bolted and the lorry drove off again and, as it rounded the top corner of the field, I caught a last glimpse of the cows, their noses frantically pressing through the wide slats in a last attempt to escape their premature execution. Tonight they'll lie on the post mortem bench.

As I walked back to the farmhouse, I saw the patch of foxgloves glowing like redhot irons on the hill, still resonating with the evening sun. It was a timely reminder that our TB problem had not been extinguished by the removal of our reactor cows from the farm, but was still very much alive and rooted in the acidity of our soils. As I walked back to the farmhouse, I remembered that the presence of foxgloves indicates high iron and high manganese levels in the soil.

*

The current approach of the UK veterinary establishment towards the control of TB remains rooted in an outmoded and uncivilized world of blanket slaughter and badly managed 'Badgerogeddons' that are naively aimed at achieving the annihilation of the TB agent from the face of the earth. Whilst livestock farms have been subjected to the mandatory measures of mass slaughter for several decades, the long-term epidemiological pattern of TB outbreaks would appear to have remained unaffected by these invasive modes of control. In stark contrast to the predictions of the most astute TB research teams, TB epidemics have continued to appear with ever-increasing frequency. The 'experts' remain privately baffled.

The problem is that their policy fails to encapsulate the most fundamental property of TB mycobacteria, which is that these agents are endemic in the open environment and can therefore never be controlled by a total wipe-out mode of control. We need to be learning how best to live alongside the TB agent and, more importantly, to be learning how best to boost our natural immunity to defend ourselves against these elusive mycobacteria. Yet despite the obvious benefits that would be gained by building up our understanding of the answers to these questions, in the UK no research has been commissioned to look at this crucial perspective of TB pathogenesis.

In the light of the fact that the incidence of this disease is currently dramatically escalating across the UK, it is high time that the Veterinary Establishment relinquishes its intransigent position on TB control. Whilst it was encouraging that Margaret Beckett, then Secretary of State for Environment, Food and Rural Affairs, repeatedly stated, 'What's the point in killing badgers if it is not going to achieve anything in the fight against TB,' it is sad that so few other people in positions of power seem to be adopting such a common-sense approach.

Last week I experienced the Pavlovian-like response of the British Veterinarian Association towards my plea to develop an investigation into an alternative 'environmental and dietary' strategy of control, as the best means of strengthening resistance to TB infection. This would not only require an about-turn in their position on the pathogenesis of TB, but also in their position on the pathogenesis of many infections — the *ironmonger* group of pathogens whose survival is totally dependent on the free iron supply in their host's tissues.

If my approach is ever shown to be correct, then it would seriously threaten the credibility of the UK Establishment's mass-slaughter programme.

I had written a letter to the editor of the Veterinary Establishment's flagship publication, which was submitted as an attempt to woo the vets away from their unilateral policy of 'overkill'. Being a letter it presented a summary version of the science surrounding the causal role of elevated iron in the food chain and how this can compromise the relevant component of our immunity, placing mammals at increased risk of contracting TB. This *high iron* facet presents an opportunity for tackling the disease. If you can influence the levels of free iron within the host, then you can control the overall outcome of the disease. The TB agent could potentially be eliminated by starving it of iron.

My letter was rapidly subjected to a burst of 'heavy vetting', and I was not surprised to receive the classic rejection for lack of scientific rigour. The irony is the editors didn't apply rigorous scientific scrutiny when reviewing the volumes of data that have been published in support of the popular 'infectious badger' theory of TB origins. The conventional consensus on TB appears to have been founded upon a series of unproven assumptions.

The Veterinary Establishment rejected the science proposed in my letter, even though it was based on hard experimental data presented by reputable international research teams. Yet despite referencing these studies, they had ignored the supporting publications and then rejected my letter on the pretext that my arguments were exclusively based on bar-stool ideas gleaned from my amateurish observations down on the farm.

In contrast, a mention of the iron-TB association to the scientific establishment in the USA is met with the totally opposite reaction. For example, when I casually mentioned my own observations of increased iron on my TB farm to a colleague at the US Environmental Protection Agency, he instantly responded by saying, 'Iron and TB – you bet. We are cleansing land of mycobacteria by directly spraying the open environment with iron microcrystals. These chelate the mycobacteria, diverting the dirty little fungal buggies into an early grave.'

In the light of the repeated failure of the badger culls to eradicate bovine TB, why on earth aren't the UK veterinary authorities paying serious attention to the positive results of the foreign studies by the Americans and Germans? Why are they resisting this alternative ray of hope?

There are some highly successful trials where TB-affected mice were treated with the iron-chelator protein lactoferrin, which reduced the incidence of TB by a hundredfold. Or the trials where lime was spread on the soil of farms infested with mycobacteria across Michigan, reducing the incidence of TB infection by tenfold as a result. These are highly impressive results, which should be taken on board by any open-minded and intelligent authority intent on designing foolproof control programmes to safeguard public and animal health. Nonetheless, the following comments sum up the Veterinary Establishment's response to my letter:

> The evidence is sometimes based on studies not directly relevant to cattle and *Mycobacterium avis*, but refers to results from *Mycobacterium avium* subspecies *paratuberculosis* (Map) and findings in mouse experiments. The inferences which are drawn from these studies and other reported data in the letter are not rigorously supported. For example, the observation that TB hotspots are all in areas where iron is mined and rainfall is high is not proven and does not explain why TB occurs elsewhere, i.e. TB is not proven to be directly correlated with soil pH or where iron is mined or where rainfall is high. Similarly there are several references to TB incidence changes over time which could be explained by a host of other factors, for example changes in the iron levels on the author's farm only proves that iron levels have changed on the farm and is at the best weak evidence of an associative link and at the worst insufficient proof of cause and effect. The communication ignores the vast scientific body of information on the epidemiology of bovine TB.

I responded to this by pointing out that I had submitted a *letter* to the editor, which was intended to alert veterinary readers to this fresh perspective on TB aetiology, and to ask the vet practices whether I could be connected to additional TB farmers in the hotspot zones in order to expand my geochemical survey.

I also informed the Veterinary Establishment that their comments were too pedantic and 'over the top' for a mere letter, particularly since they had implied that I ought to be providing a full spectrum of hard evidence within my first letter on this subject to the academic literature.

Whilst the reviewers had correctly raised the issue that hotspots of TB are not always sited in areas where iron mining has existed (albeit only two areas that I can see), their comment had failed to grasp the prerequisite of the theory, 'elevated iron in the bovine food chain'. This can arise in various contexts where iron ore beds are not sufficiently concentrated in local bedrock to justify the economic mining of the ore, but where, nonetheless, iron is still highly concentrated in topsoils for a variety of other geochemical reasons. I had pointed out the striking correlation between the iron mining areas and TB hotspot zones, and then utilized this as a means of providing a general yardstick for demonstrating that the high iron factor offered a plausible explanation for the distribution of TB incidence across the UK.

Their argument here is flawed because where there are a number of variable factors contributing to the animal's iron status and if only one factor is altered then this may not be critical. By the same token I realize that finding an association between iron hotspots and TB does not prove that high iron causes clinical TB. There are always going to be different environmental influences that will bring about exactly the same end effect of elevated iron within the biosystem, which in turn will influence the outcome of any TB infection in the same way.

For example, use of the anti-lactoferrin insecticide wormer Levamisole is currently very prevalent on UK livestock farms where it is used in various drench or systemic pour-on wormer formulations. Although exposure to this molecule will initially create an acceleration in the synthesis of the immune protein lactoferrin, boosting the immune system, the long-term repercussions of such an exposure are going to be a bit like driving a car at full throttle throughout its entire life. You will burn the car out, driving it prematurely to the scrapyard. In this respect the long-term effect of exposures to Levamisole causes a reduction of lactoferrin secretion due to the disrupting effects of this chemical at its target receptors on T-lymphocyte immune cells, e.g. the receptors that mediate the secretion of lactoferrin. This reduction represents a well-known toxicological mechanism by which a receptor can adapt to a toxic insult, by becoming sensitized and/or reducing the rate at which receptors are replenished. The net effect is a long-term, perhaps permanent deficiency in the secretion of lactoferrin, which in the context of this study brings about a markedly decreased level of immunity to TB infection.

Lactoferrin is an immune protein that is a component of exocrine secretions. It is manufactured in the epithelia of the gut, lungs and tear ducts, and in granulocytes where it is used as an iron chelator and antioxidant in the armoury of immune defence against invading pathogens. Lactoferrin performs a pivotal role in the defence against invading TB, where it competes against the mycobacteria for the supply of free iron within the tissues, ultimately 'ironing out' the lifeblood of the TB agent.

Therefore the simultaneous exposure of mammals to high iron food chains and anti-lactoferrin toxic agents (e.g. the pesticide wormer) could be sufficient to raise the levels of free iron in the tissues to a threshold, which is ripe for a TB takeover.

Whilst I understand the reviewer's point that the elevation of iron on my own TB-affected farm doesn't supply hard evidence to substantiate the theory, my letter didn't actually attempt to do this. In the light of the published experimental evidence on high iron and TB infection, I had indicated that these observations on my own and other farms could turn out to be extremely important, and were sufficient to warrant expansion to a full-scale comparative geo-chemical investigation covering all of the main TB regions across the UK.

I feel that mainstream journals ought to be publishing the plausible creative leaps in scientific thinking, rather than rejecting them outright. For the history of science has repeatedly shown that most of the advancement within Academe has stemmed from intuitive sparks of insight, often originating from the layperson. Yet whenever these ideas have been successfully suppressed by the mainstream in the past due to peer prejudice, or commercial or political pressures, the evolution of scientific knowledge suffered a setback as a result.

Consider the negative outcome for medicine if Jenner's original radical observations on the immunization of milkmaids against smallpox had been rejected outright at the start. Jenner's initial observations were based on a group of milk maidens who were working with cowpox-infected cattle in a cowshed on a single farm in Gloucestershire. The milkmaids had unwittingly immunized themselves against smallpox as a result. If Jenner's hypothesis had been blocked on grounds that his initial observations were only made on a single farm and therefore could not be shown to hold true for every milkmaid operating across the UK then his important discovery may never have been accepted.

I also take issue with the Veterinary Establishment when they state that the arguments in my letter were not based on rigorous scientific studies. Whilst my own analytical studies to date clearly provide a limited amount of hard evidence, I feel that their comments are inappropriate in respect of the validity of the data, which was referenced in my letter. The huge funding for badger cull trials is not based upon hard evidence or even mediocre supporting evidence – the evidence is contradictory. Instead, the funding is being used to carry out extensive trials to provide evidence to answer the question. To ask me for the quality and scope of evidence obtained at the end of such trials at the start of my investigation is nonsense.

If you have read the veterinary critique above, I should point out that my letter had clearly indicated that these experiments had involved mice rather than bovines, and *Mycobacterium paratuberculosis* rather than *Mycobacterium tuberculosis*. This is the appropriate and usual way of doing scientific research – you start small with pilot studies and scale up when and if things look promising. The research with mice was presumably felt worthwhile originally or it would not have received funding. Furthermore, I cannot see how the differences between the species and strains involved in these experiments should fundamentally weaken the overall relevance of these trials to the context of bovine TB outbreaks in the UK.

My letter had also pointed out that all strains of *Mycobacterium* require a source of iron to manifest their pathogenicity, irrespective of whether the *M. paratuberculosis* or *M. tuberculosis* strain is involved. I was particularly annoyed over their failure to recognize the potential relevance of the positive study in which the number of TB pathogens in infected mice had been reduced a hundredfold after treatment with the iron chelator lactoferrin. The Veterinary Establishment had rejected this valuable research on the basis that the work relates to TB in mice and not TB in bovines.

These reviewers must be aware of the universal use of unfortunate lab mice in millions of drug-licensing trials where animal reaction to pharmaceutical exposure is exploited as a best means of assessing the potential health effects of those chemicals upon human beings. Furthermore, the entire global establishment has heralded the results of the mice studies carried out by Dr Moira Bruce at Edinburgh as a plausible means of proving the causal connection between human consumption of BSE-affected cow tissues and the development of variant CJD in humans. Moira Bruce's conclusions were in support of the prevailing 'politically correct' theory at that time.

Once again, it seems that the work of outsider scientists has to be complete and proven before it is funded. A good example of pathological prejudice against 'outsiders' was enacted via the peer-review system operated by *The Veterinary Record* journal. One of my own papers on TSEs was rejected in 2004 due to 'lack of scientific rigour', despite having presented some ground-breaking data from the analyses of 200 soil and antler samples, which I'd collected across chronic wasting disease cluster zones in the USA and Canada.

Ironically, a few weeks later, a depressingly dull and unoriginal paper by Chihota et al., from the prestigious Compton Labs in the

UK, had attempted to counter a misrepresented version of my paper and data. The paper was published by *The Veterinary Record*, despite the admission by the author that they couldn't afford to carry out any analyses – 'to carry out blood testing and analysis on the necessary scale would have been prohibitively expensive. Instead, we sent a questionnaire survey to farmers asking them what minerals were deficient in their area and compared this with data from the National Soil Inventory.'

Well, next time I'll know not to pay for the expensive analysis and I'll make do with an anecdotal questionnaire like the experts!

Back on the TB battle front, the British Veterinary Establishment's rejection of the widely recognized 'high iron' perspective of TB pathogenesis betrays their determination to remain wedded to the current slaughter strategy. These uncivilized strategies of mass slaughter are by no means exclusive to the control of TB. They have been repeatedly implemented over the last century to suppress the outbreaks of supposedly 'infectious' diseases, for example the TSEs.

It is sad to witness such a penchant for the mass murder of animals. Surely, it is the duty of any responsible authority to try to provide a more civilized option of disease control before resorting to mass slaughter? The badger myth surrounding TB control has now infected the rural community to the extent that vigilante groups have been taking the law into their own hands and illegally gassing the badgers in the TB areas. I was appalled to learn that one of these cyanide sessions had taken place on my own farm, at the most vibrant badger set in our valley. The badgers had become the target of a moonlight gas attack by a bunch of goons, who apart from anything were so careless that they forgot to take the empty gas bottles away. I had found the cylinders slumped across a patch of bluebells adjoining the set the next morning. If only these insensitive idiots had been aware that the bluebell bulbs provide the dietary source of concentrated iron that enables a TB infection to take hold in the animals. These badger bashers would have carried out a more effective job if they'd uprooted the bluebell bulbs and left the poor old badgers alone.

But perhaps the most positive piece of news from behind the iron curtain of the TB hazard zone involves the results of some pilot studies I had conducted on a batch of 'inconclusive' TB-reactor cows on my farm. I had intensively fed these cows with a mineral-protein formulation that was designed to chelate the iron and also to impair the uptake of iron into the cow. I was running this pilot experiment with the aim of starving the TB organism to death. The results so far have been encouraging, involving six inconclusive animals on my farm (five were milking cows) that had been fed the formulation during each milking over a one-month period. At the TB test last week, the government vets decreed that four out of the five treated animals had recovered and reverted to TB-free status, whilst the remaining one had retained her TB 'inconclusive' status. The sixth TB inconclusive animal, which was a beef steer and had never been fed the formulation, was found to have progressed to full 'TB reactor' status and is committed to slaughter.

Whilst the positive results of this pilot study are not significant in scientific terms, because of the small numbers of animals involved, they indicate the likelihood that these 'inconclusive' cattle are no longer reacting to the TB test because they had been treated with a feed which chelates and competes for the iron. It is imperative that this investigation is advanced to the next stage and tested on a much larger group of animals.

Farewell

by Nigel Purdey

The last time I saw Mark in good health was under the Camberwell railway arches on a warm October evening. We'd just come back from researching in Kent during the Indian summer of 2005. I was buying a new tyre before the arch garage closed, whilst Mark had nipped into the pub across the road for a pee. I explained the bus route over to Hammersmith, as I always did, helped him on with his bulging rucksack and said goodbye.

The next time we spoke he was having problems with his health. He'd begun to get odd symptoms whilst playing the sax at a gig, noticing that the sound would trigger tinnitus and problems with spatial coordination. He'd gone to his GP, thinking that it might be an unusual virus, and was given some blood tests, which all came back normal. He was told he was probably fine. Over the next few weeks he got worse and went back to his GP, who gave him some more tests, which again came back normal and nothing more was done. He later wrote about this period:

> During the days before Christmas, I had developed some bizarre neuro-psychiatric symptoms involving flashing lights, loss of left-sided sensation, poor 3D orientation, migraines, a ringing sound in my head, vomiting, photophobia which culminated in the total loss of use of my legs, an inability to dress, to put on my boots and, eventually, to communicate with others.
>
> The onset of my syndrome was most ironic in that these symptoms had first kicked in whilst I was writing a chapter for my book on the clinical profile of victims of variant CJD.

Strangely enough, my GP had even put me down as a possible case of CJD. For example, one particularly humiliating incident had seen me get down from the tractor and collapse onto a field that was 6 in deep in mud. I had to crawl on my belly with my legs sprawled out, like a frog negotiating a surface of ice, then lever my body across two fields of mud to get back to the farmhouse. At one point I had to scale a barbed wire fence and found myself pivoted along my belly by the barbed wire. I hung there for a while like a World War One soldier escaping the trenches.

Some of my cows were standing across the field and had sensed a problem and started ambling towards me. One of them approached me and was obviously bewildered by the sight of my body bizarrely strung up over the barbed wire. She stared deeply and earnestly into my eyes. This reminded me of the time when I was treating one of my BSE cows with a sulphate molecule to try to cure her of BSE. Just before I administered the injection the cow had engaged with me in an identical mode of eye contact and this reminded me of the stern words of a neighbouring farmer, who had insisted that it was cruel to keep the cow alive for my own selfish experimental interests. He was right, and my intensive eye contact with this cow whilst I was pivoted along the barbed wire fence had taken me back to this incident, particularly pertinent since I was now suffering from a brain disease myself. The incident had detonated deep in my memory and stirred up my feelings of guilt.

Mark's health got still worse and when he went back to the surgery for a third time he saw the other practice GP, who immediately sent him to Taunton Hospital for a brain scan. He was now having difficulty walking, but managed to make it into the hospital, with a little help from Margaret, and have the scan.

I had started to suspect a brain tumour and this was confirmed after an MRI scan at Musgrove Hospital and the operation at Frenchay. A massive astro-glioma multiforme grade 4 malignant tumour was found in my right parietal/occipital lobe — interestingly, this represents the area of the brain involved with abstract thinking (a well-worn area with me, maybe!). The tumour was compressing my brain to such an extent that it had been causing the life-threatening symptoms which I'd been experiencing. I now realize that it may have been growing for years.

We now had to wait for an appointment to come through for an operation at Frenchay Hospital in Bristol. It was the weekend and, as we feared, nothing seemed to be happening. Many questions were flooding through our minds. Why was it taking so long to get an appointment? Perhaps they couldn't operate? Perhaps there was an admin oversight and the scans had got mislaid?

As the weekend went on Mark deteriorated rapidly, becoming less articulate, nauseous and tired. His body was gradually stiffening and his conversation changed in tone. He was searching for comforting memories and images and wanted us to bring in some special items — there was the photograph of mum and dad on a style at Little Hadham and an anthology of poems from school called 'Voices'. He talked a lot about various friends — how John would come in to his cottage in the winter and with a great flourish unwind the longest multicoloured home-knitted scarf in the world. And then there were the old walks in places filled with powerful memories and recollections of happy times. He was bathing himself in warm, heart-centred memories and I found it almost unbearable to watch because he was dealing with his mortality — unflinching.

On Saturday afternoon a nurse finally told Margaret and myself that the tumour was very deep inside the brain, just above the brainstem and they may not be able to operate. This was devastating news. Exactly a year ago my sister's neighbour had died very quickly of three brainstem tumours. His doctors couldn't do anything for him. I got on the net that evening and poured over PubMed to find anything that might give us some hope if the brainstem tumour was confirmed.

At last, on Monday afternoon, a doctor came in with the scans. We were, in a sense, relieved to see a tumour just under the skull, which was accessible to surgery. Nevertheless it was huge and awesome and it shook me up just thinking about it inside Mark's brain. Later that afternoon Mark went up to Frenchay in the ambulance in preparation for the operation first thing in the morning.

It's a miracle that a stranger can walk in from the street with some obscure neurological problem and find such a high degree of first rate nursing care and neuro-surgery shortly after arrival. Since the patients seldom ever return to their wards after their discharge from the hospital, it seems unfair that these professionals rarely get to witness the successful outcome of their brilliant work. The brain surgery at Frenchay, which uses advanced computer modelling of the tumour, removed 95% of the 80 mm diameter malignant tissue during a protracted operation carried out on the longest, darkest winter night of 2005 – at the winter solstice. It was a spiritual heal as well as a physical heal, as all of my neurological and psychiatric faculties have rapidly returned to near normal since arriving back on my farm. Like many near death encounters, my whole life was presented to me during the operation, when I was better able to understand my tumour, as well as see options for the future, regarding how best to deal with the problem.

It was a very tense day in which we walked back and forth between the canteen and the ward, waiting, drinking endless coffee and asking for news of the operation. I was in the corridor, when I saw a trolley coming out of the operating theatre and, feeling sure it was Mark, I approached. I was shaking as I looked into the eyes of the person on the trolley. I said 'Hi, Mark, how are you?' He replied, upbeat as ever, 'Hi Nige, ya, I'm OK.' That was good enough for me, he was still with us. We sat with him as he slowly unwound. I made a joke about the Scottish mineral water being rather low in magnesium and he laughed and made a good quip back. I was relieved because I felt the old Mark was very much here, emerging from the trauma of surgery and after-affects of the drugs. He later told us about his fear during and after the operation. He thought he'd possibly been in a massive car crash and was unsure about whether he was in hospital or taking part in some secret experiment.

One of the other things he spoke about on that first afternoon was an intense spiritual experience he'd had during surgery, which had helped him come to terms with his mortality. Coming through the trauma he said he had no fear of death – although he didn't want to die at all.

All fears that I had about my possible forthcoming death during the operation were relinquished when I focused on a mantra, which I'd been given as a 19-year-old when I did a crash course in transcendental meditation in Cork. My sounding of the mantra enabled me to home into the essence of what I would call the Holy Spirit, which was surprisingly abundant in that operating room. This provided me with the option for a future of eternal life. The choice was mine, and I felt instantly energized by the experience, losing my fear and negativity over what was happening. I managed to transcend the guilt about my past, which had possibly played a role in the cause of the tumour, and I felt healed.

Amazingly, despite the fact that I hadn't been interviewed by BBC radio for several years, an old broadcast covering one of my interviews was being aired on the world service just as I was knocked out with the anaesthetic. My voice had also awoken a spiritual healer friend of mine from her sleep, alerting her to my ordeal, and my instant requirement for spiritual healing.

The crude rate of brain cancer in 2003 in the UK was 8.4 cases in men and 6 cases in women per 100,000 population. There appears to be a slight rise in their incidence over the last 30 years. The glioblastoma multiforme grade 4 is a right bugger of a primary tumour, which originates in the brain cells rather than spreading from elsewhere. Being grade 4 it was the most aggressive type and the prognosis was not very good – the average life expectancy being about a year from diagnosis. But there are a few long-term survivors, and it's well worth being positive and seeking out everything on offer – we were determined to do this.

The standard treatment is surgery, followed by radiotherapy, sometimes combined with chemotherapy. Most of the chemo has bad side-effects and may not give much additional life expectancy and many patients opt for quality of life, foregoing the chemo.

When I was released from the hospital, they gave me a freebie wheelchair as a Christmas present. This made me assume, albeit incorrectly, that I was supposed to be a cripple for the rest of my life, and it instantly cracked me up into tears. I thought of the times that I'd walked out of buildings and institutions with my family, when we would be heading away on holidays or walks in the hills, but this time it was different. According to expert predictions I was never expected to walk again on my own – but the miracles continued. When we arrived back home at High Barn Farm, we left the wheelchair folded in the back of the car and I found myself walking into my home unaided, which was weird because I hadn't walked for many days. By Christmas morning, I started dancing to my daughter's CD of Celtic music on our kitchen floor. By Boxing Day afternoon, I was walking across the tops of the smooth boulders along the Lee Abbey seafront, my favourite refuge on the west Somerset coastline. My eternal gratitude is also extended to my tight knit group of family and friends who rapidly rallied a strong team of support to help my wife Margaret cope with the farm and our multitude of children during the crisis.

I soon started researching potential treatments for brain tumours and was heartened by how much was going on in the field.

Perhaps the leading experimental treatment involves the genetically modified herpes virus, HSV-1, which is injected into the brain, adjacent to the tumour. The virus is engineered to feed solely on tumour cells and dies when it runs out of tumour. This is currently in the final stage of trials.

Another experimental treatment involves the intravenous injections of an attenuated strain of a chicken virus, Newcastle disease virus. Both of these sound horrendous, but they're achieving quite good success with few side-effects.

I came across a couple of interesting aspirin-based drug approaches for brain tumours. One, which is still experimental, involves Farnesyl thiosalicylic acid, which inhibits a cancer cell proliferation protein called Ras. The other is called sulfasalazine, which is already licensed for arthritis, and has recently showed potential in treating brain tumours.

I'd recommend a look at Ben Williams's story. A long-term survivor and psychology professor, he gives a lot of detail about the conventional and complementary therapies he has used over the years. You can read his story on Al Musella's excellent brain tumour website, where you can also find video lectures, other survivor stories and a wide variety of research information.

There are many complementary dietary approaches for treating cancer. One that particularly caught my attention involves various mushrooms such as shitaki, reishi, maitaki, *Coriolus versicolor*, *Cordyceps*, *Agaricus blazei*, *Phellinus linteus* and *P. pini*. They contain molecules which have been shown to have some benefit in treating cancer and are part of mainstream treatments in some Asian countries. In one experiment I found that the *Phellinus* varieties achieved 97% and 100% respectively in killing cancer cells in vitro – unfortunately this doesn't necessarily translate to in vivo, but there were a few papers showing success in treating human cancers. White tea is another interesting substance currently undergoing research, which contains higher concentrations of the active polyphenols than the more widely researched and touted green tea – it tastes good too.

Mark soon became interested in what had caused his tumour.

Whilst my self-destructive mismanagement of stress and anger in my life had possibly played a role in the cause of my tumour, I have now started looking for a common environmental factor, which is present in the homes of all of the victims of gliomas in my region of west Somerset. My preliminary enquiries into this cluster of cases came up with the presence of copper deposits from hot water boilers in the victims' residences. The intensity of copper from our own ancient back boiler had clearly made me extremely hypersensitive to the water during the time of my acute illness. Perhaps the bonding of the copper into the tumour tissues in the brain explained why I had become sensitive to electro-magnetic fields. I spent hours every day in front of my computer screen. The copper may have acted as a conduit for this energy, perhaps initiating radical chain reactions, which mutated DNA in the copper-contaminated tissues – in my case, within the parietal lobe.

Considering the rarity of brain cancer there does seem to be a lot in the tiny villages around Mark. But its not really clear what lies behind this. Mark was interested in copper as a possible cause, but there are other factors that may be relevant. About a year prior to his diagnosis the hilltop radio mast, which is 1 kilo-metre away from the farm over open fields, was converted to a tetra system. There are two other tetra masts nearby and there is research linking tetra systems to cancer. He'd been building an extension in 2004/5, which, because he was working outside, would have given him more potential exposure to the tetra micro-waves.

There were other possible scenarios, such as bangs on the head which he'd sustained in the milking parlour and at Nettlecombe church. He'd had some fires on the farm in which he burnt old fencing and treated timbers and had got a bit careless about breathing in the smoke. Perhaps the most likely explanation might be that his research work in contaminated zones, such as Guam, Colorado and Italy, involved him in handling samples, some of which were radioactive.

There were many possible factors but in the end we just don't know for certain what caused his cancer.

> I appear to have transformed the negativity of my operation into a positive revolution in many aspects of my life, such as my relationships, general psychological and physical health. It has left me empowered.
>
> I remain optimistic for recovery and that the good nutrition, love, prayers and peace provided by so many of my friends and family will enable me to inhibit future proliferation of malignant cells.

Alas, Mark only lived another ten months after writing this. He was up and down for much of this time. He had fits, most of which were quite small, but on one occasion he had to go into hospital because of a build-up of pressure in the brain and he got no treatment for hours. Margaret realized that all he needed was some extra steroids to bring down the swelling, but despite constantly badgering the staff nothing happened and he got worse. Eventually a nurse gave him the steroids and he started improving. Unfortunately, after this incident he started to lose his sight and he was eventually told that he had atrophy of the optic nerve. This was almost certainly caused by the swelling of the brain, which squashed and deprived the optic nerve of oxygen during that day at the hospital. As a result he became virtually blind, which just added another burden to his life.

He agreed to have radiotherapy treatment, which went quite well, and by midsummer the scans showed that the tumour hadn't regrown after the therapy. Sometimes when we talked on the phone I felt I was talking to the old Mark. We joked and had long heated debates, like in the old days, about his theory and his intention to do more work on bovine TB. His long-term memory was good and he still had command over many scientific concepts, but his short-term memory had really suffered. I was constantly bowled over by his optimism about his health, and whilst not wanting to knock him back I didn't really share it. The survival figures were just very poor and I guessed that it might be difficult to get onto one of the experimental treatments because there might not be a vacancy when needed or he might not be well enough to participate.

He tried some acupuncture and Chinese herbs and had a few supplements. We cleaned up his environment and modified his diet, but he decided not to go all out for an experimental treatment, and spent as much quality time as possible with his family.

In May our mother sadly died rather unexpectedly of pancreatic cancer and Mark and his family came up to Much Hadham, where mum had continued to live next door to the Red House. This enabled him to reconnect with all the powerful places of his youth such as the Rib Valley, and we took some of the old walks around the village.

Then two months later our paternal Aunt, who lived near Mark, also sadly died and this stirred up some problems that we'd been facing over her life and relationships. Although Mark and his family had been on good terms with her and had seen her quite often in the past, she seemed to have slowly turned against all our family and instead — for some reason — was virtually worshipping her neighbours, who we feared would inherit her estate. Mark couldn't go to the funeral because he was tied in knots by these issues, which dated back over the decades of their relationship.

In the late summer a scan showed that not only had the tumour regrown in the same part of the brain, but it had also spread to the frontal lobe. It was the size of a tennis ball and must have grown incredibly fast over a few weeks. Chemo was suggested but I think we all knew that it wasn't going to achieve much, and might make life worse with the side-effects. Enrolling in an experimental viral trial had problems mainly because of the size of the tumour and it had to be faced that perhaps he wasn't up to these kinds of aggressive therapy.

In October Mark started to go downhill and it was clear that Margaret was facing a huge challenge herself and was going to need quite a bit of help to look after both him and the children. My sister, Ginny, and I started to come down for a few days at a time to help out. Several neighbours, old school friends and two council carers also helped out during the last few weeks.

A plethora of devices arrived at the farm to help with Mark's mobility – a hoist, ramps, grab-rails, adjustable chairs, a hospital bed and a special mattress. Some of these gadgets were not that well designed and we soon came up with a host of new inventions and modifications. We had all discovered a liking for the TV programme *Dragon's Den* and we tested out our new ideas in our crazy version of the show, which kept us going during this difficult time.

One of my roles as a male was to assist in catheter duty, of the slip-on variety. One day Margaret, who'd been checking out Mark's emails, said there'd only been one, offering the usual discounted viagra, and she'd deleted it confident that Mark wasn't interested. At that precise moment I was having difficulty in performing the intricate and crucial manoeuvre of slipping the catheter over a rather dejected penis and I commented that perhaps she should have taken up the offer as it might have proved rather useful in our current predicament. We had a good laugh about this and at least got some endorphins flowing if nothing else.

Music as always reached deep into Mark's body and soul and we tried a range of old favourite jazz and folk CDs and even bought a record player from ebay to play some of his large vinyl collection. Mark's foot tapped, a smile broke out and his body came to life as he responded to the pulse of Joshua Redmond's furious railing solo, which swept the rafters of the barn. 'Who's this Nige?' If he asked who it was then you knew it had hit the spot.

His old school friend Robb came over from Ireland for a few days to help out. Even when Mark was too tired to join in with spoken contributions Robb and I tried talking to each other about things we'd done with Mark in such a way that he would feel included. We were playing to his gallery and every so often we would see a smile of recognition forming on his face.

I tried adapting the kind of Haileyburian parade-ground commands, which would usually crack Mark up, to introduce some levity into the daily routines, particularly standing up for the changing of trousers etc. Mark was quite stiff and weak and it was tricky to get him standing and supported on his frame. I issued commands like a demented sergeant major from school: 'Squad, staaand up. Squad schhhhtion. Wait for it Purdey, stand eeeeasy.' Margaret did the honours with the changing. On a particularly grim afternoon Margaret and I sat in the bedroom whilst the GP, Dr Philip, examined Mark to assess whether he was well enough to go for an appointment to the hospital to discuss chemo. It wasn't looking good and Dr Philip had the very difficult task of telling Mark that he didn't think he was up to it and, by implication, not up to receiving the treatment. It was a chilling and heartbreaking moment as Mark took this in. He nodded, understanding and just looked downwards and blinked. Margaret held his hand. He was effectively being told that there was nothing else that could be done.

Mark kept up a brave face and wasn't too deterred; the plan was to stay on at home rather than go into hospital or a hospice and see how things went. Three weeks before he died some friends took him down to give an interview at the local radio station, 10Radio, in Wiveliscombe. For an hour and a quarter he answered questions about his research interspersed with some musical recordings he'd made with local musicians.

Mark died peacefully, just after lunch, on Remembrance Sunday, 12 November 2006, 48 years to the day after the dedicatee of this book. It was a cruel irony that he was taken so young by a disease that was so closely related to what he'd spent much of his life researching. One only has to read the many tributes on his website to see the depth of affection and admiration in which he was held. In the end of course we still have his ideas, which live on encapsulated in his writings and the films which I made with him.

Over the course of his illness he remained resolutely optimistic and showed incredible courage in the face of darkness. In his life he came from a position of zero power as an outsider and a layman and yet he managed to infiltrate the upper echelons of the scientific world and get them to sit up and listen to his ideas. He had no time for the dithering empty words of twittering bureaucracy or the inertia of the status quo. He was totally committed to his endeavour to shift a paradigm – a virtually impossible task for even the most established scientist.

He believed, as I do, that there is a survival of the spirit after death and I like to think he's just slipped through the net of our world into one of the many other dimensions of which the universe is comprised. One thing's for sure – he's bound to have a theory about it.

Don't let the buggers get you down

by Nigel Purdey

There are many myths surrounding Mark's life. Was there really a campaign of dirty tricks directed against him or was he just paranoid and looking at events through his own tinted specs? At first, I didn't know what to make of all the stories he told me of negative events. My initial instincts were that they were probably just coincidence. But whilst the first half dozen weird events could be put down to chance, by the time I'd counted 20 or so, I was starting to change my mind and became convinced that something was going on. Whilst some incidents probably had a simple explanation, the continuous intensity of the others understandably must have made him prone to a degree of paranoia. And yet he could nearly always manage to step back and laugh at himself over the craziness of it all.

One of the features that clinched it for me was the way in which the events would occur for several years and then everything would go quiet for a few years. Mark would say the change seemed to track the change of Agriculture Minister. I concluded that if Mark had been paranoid then he would always have been finding some malign significance in ordinary events and there would not have been these prolonged 'off' periods when he said nothing occurred.

Margaret, Mark's wife, said that it was very difficult for her to accept that something was amiss because of the implications that it had for their family life. It was too depressing and frightening to accept that one was living one's life under the scrutiny of a bunch of criminals, whose sole intent was to shut you up.

The incidents took the form of classic dirty tricks. There was phone-tapping, which was evident on the many occasions when we spoke, from the buzzing, whirring, clicking and the line eventually going dead. This seemed to be activated by key words such as organophosphates, prion or BSE, which I gather is how this sort of thing works. Then there was the 48-hour phone block, which would always occur after he'd been in the news. You would phone the farm repeatedly and get a normal ring tone, but no one would answer, so you didn't report a fault. Finally, after 48 hours you would get through (it was usually at 11 a.m.) and Mark would say that he'd been in, waiting for calls, but the phone hadn't rung for two days. Friends and relatives all reported the same experience. After two days any journalist following up the story would have given up.

But we hit back from time to time with our own brand of mischievous counter-disinformation, designed to worry our eavesdroppers. One of the more extreme plans I hatched was for us to discuss on the phone some spoof redhot pesticide and prion research, which had been conducted by a fictitious Eastern bloc scientist (with an untraceable name). We would make the info rather vague so that our friends would chase around trying to identify the individual and his lab, but would not be put off when they drew a blank. The plan was for Mark to meet this scientist, probably played by myself (budget wouldn't run to a proper actor), in a London park café. The dress code was standard 'spy' – shabby macs, dark glasses, copy of a John le Carré novel for identification. The basic plan was to chat over a coffee and see if either any suspicious looking men were peeping at us from behind a newspaper or there were any buggers lurking in the bushes with their shotgun mikes. Unfortunately we only discussed this on the phone, as a wind-up, and never went all the way through with the plan because it would have been too time consuming, but it relieved the tension and gave us a small sense of power. O happy days!

Mark told me that the mail was occasionally tampered with – there would be nothing for weeks and then a large brown envelope would arrive with all the mail inside, and some of it would have been opened.

There were many unusual, time-wasting, bizarre and sometimes dangerous individuals who made contact. They would turn up out of the blue and usually force their presence on the family, and would often be found rifling through the farm stores and out-buildings – pushy types who you couldn't get rid of. Mark suspected that some of these characters had actually bugged the farm, but he never had any evidence of this. We did all agree, in retrospect, that some of these characters might well have been just sad, eccentric individuals, rather than the evil agents of a faceless conspiracy.

One supposed journalist, Alistair, who contacted me as well as Mark and sounded vaguely plausible at first, had us running scared for a couple of weeks with his brand of conspiratorial mayhem. He told me that Mark should go into hiding because a local campaigner was out to get him. There was an eventual showdown in which Alistair, following an assault he'd committed with a pitchfork at another farm, came to Mark's farm and threatened him. Alistair had forgotten to mention that he was the dangerous one. The police were called and he was eventually sectioned.

The fact that these sorts of things went on doesn't prove that Mark was correct in his theory; it shows that 'they' acknowledged he had influence and the potential to damage their interests. He had a powerful pen and a voice that was heard from Harvard to Glastonbury via numerous village halls. Any person with his kind of views, who gains an audience with Ministers and other influential people, would be considered a threat.

But what lay behind these events? I'd probably subscribe to the explanation of cock-up or genuine ignorance. Where TSEs are concerned, these were new, complex diseases and we didn't know much about them. It was on the cards that some recent change in farming practice or contamination might have been the cause. Indeed, changes in rendering techniques were initially blamed. The truth could turn out to be very dangerous for the Government, as they might turn out to be liable.

Alternatively, perhaps some studies were undertaken in the early years of BSE by a select few, which were not published due to the results being too damning of a government department. Then again, perhaps all Mark's problems stemmed from his pesticide work. Most academic researchers in this field are quite low key and didn't get news coverage. Mark was different. He blitzed the media with his ideas and he would have proved a sharp thorn in the side of this very powerful industry. We never had any hard evidence of who was behind the campaign but I know Mark certainly had his strong suspicions.

The testing of pesticides in the early days was limited in its scope. No one knew what their subtle long-term affects would be. There was no thought given to the susceptibility of individuals who have weaknesses in detoxification enzymes and who would be more likely to develop long-term damage from exposure. We knew about OP's anti-cholinesterase activity and their mutagenicity, but not much else. We didn't know about their epigenetic affects or adduction or the many interactions they have with other proteins. The general trend in pesticide licensing and use over the last 50 years has been gradually more restrictive, with outright banning of some pesticides, subtle phasing out of others, reduction of maximum doses and increases in protective measures. If we'd got the testing correct at the start we wouldn't have seen this trend, and maybe we're still not at the end of this trend.

The instigators of dirty tricks are fortunate because they can easily play to the pathological inertia amongst opinion formers to accept anything with a whiff of conspiracy. It's almost a conditioned reflex within the chattering classes. How often do you hear the retort, 'I'm not the type of person to believe in conspiracy theories.' You cannot disabuse this type of person of this received wisdom. Where there is an agreement between two or more persons to break the law at some time in the future, surely not that rare an event, conspiracies exist. The trouble is that there are some tiresome and daft theories around, which give conspiracies a bad name and spoil it for the rest of us!

Mark gave interviews to a number of journalists in the mid-nineties and I've used two of these, Bob Woffinden's in the *Guardian* and Brigid McConville's in the *Times*, to put together the next section, together with my own recollection of talks I had with him over the years.

Mark summed up his experiences like this:

> For 18 years now, I have found my work and personal integrity subjected to a steady trickle of derisory ridicule and dirty tricks. During the 1980s my farm and family became the victims of a succession of 'once in a lifetime' type physical disasters, including arson, firearm intimidation, vandalism of my research library and communications, insidious infiltration by a bizarre array of bogus Greens, phoney freelance journalists, cutting of the phone line, phone-tapping, the 48 hour phone block after I'd been in the news or had a film out, and mail interference. There were honey trap scenarios, such as the seductive approach by a scantily clad pseudo-student from the Leeds Tech college, who was supposedly doing a dissertation on my theory. After becoming suspicious, my investigations revealed that she was not registered at the college.
>
> It invariably transpired that the true objectives of these 'agent provocateurs' was either subtly to set about discrediting my social and scientific esteem or to find out the current state of play of my research or wear me and my family down. Once my work gained support from the likes of the former Minister of Defence, Tom King, and HRH the Prince of Wales, the physical aspects of this harassment abruptly ceased.

The start of the troubles for Mark began one morning in 1984 when a MAFF official appeared at his caravan door, instructing him to comply with the Warble Fly Treatment Order of 1982. 'She said we were in a zone where it was compulsory for us to treat our cows with a systemic organophosphate warble fly treatment, called phosmet. It was as if my whole life became focused. Prior to that, I thought I knew what was happening in the farming industry. The propaganda put out by the chemical companies is enormous, and so I was concerned, but I hadn't started actively campaigning at that stage.'

MAFF adamantly refuted the suggestion that there could be a danger from the OP treatment to humans or cattle. Besides phosmet, the animals were potentially subject to a plethora of other OP treatments, such as worming boluses, lice and parasite controls, fly-sprays, insecticide-laced ear-tags, and even a cocktail of residues in the feed. Incredibly, the officially recommended method of disposing of surplus sheep dip was to spread it over pasture. Humans, of course, in addition to administering the treatments had their own additional exposures in their environment.

Mark had no alternative but to fight the Order in the courts and Mr Justice Stocker found in his favour. The case got him national publicity in the press and on TV and he appeared triumphantly on BBC2's *Out of Court* with his solicitor Peter Ward, whose expertise had made the victory possible.

In late 1984 mad cow disease or BSE first occurred in cattle in the UK, but it wasn't fully identified until two years later. BSE is one of the diseases involving an abnormal form of a common protein found in the brain and nervous system, called the prion. As time went on, Mark noticed that the incidence of BSE closely followed the usage of the phosmet anti-warble treatment. He was aware of some work by Dr James Hope of the AFRC neuropathogenesis unit at Edinburgh, in which he refers to the fact that the structural surface of the prion protein mimics that of cholinesterase. This suggested that a molecule that targets cholinesterase (like OPs) may well target the prion – and so could underlie BSE.

Mark cultivated several international contacts and one of these, Professor Satoshi Ishikawa, a Japanese expert on OP pesticides, wrote to him saying, 'Your description linking mad cows to orga-nophosphates is exactly true.' But Mark wanted to test his theory and he was given the opportunity when one of his own cows, Damson (bought in from a chemically run farm), developed BSE.

> Before calling in the Ministry, I blood-tested her. It was probably illegal, because once you suspect BSE you must report it. The red blood cell enzyme acetylcholinesterase was down by about 20% in Damson, compared with three control cows. This wasn't proof that it was OP poisoning, but it did suggest that OP inhibition of cholinesterase could be involved in the biochemistry of the disease.
>
> I wanted to treat her with an oxime and atropine that Professor Ishikawa had recommended. My vet, Christopher Budge, man-aged to get hold of some from the Musgrove Hospital in Taunton where it had been stockpiled in case Saddam Hussein had used nerve gases in the first Gulf War. We injected Damson with oxime and atropine sulphate and within 90 minutes we got a dramatic remission of symptoms. We wanted to treat her over a six-month period but it was a hopelessly uneconomic, unrealistic aim, although it would have been a scientific trial, albeit preliminary.

Budge told the *Independent* newspaper, 'If I can help to clarify his theory, I am happy to do so.' He sent some BSE brain material off to a colleague at Cambridge for analysis to check this out. Tragically, a few weeks later he was killed outside Taunton when his car veered into the path of an oncoming lorry. A headline in the local paper, a few weeks later, read 'Riddle of vet's car on lorry's side of road.' Then 'The Minehead inquest heard that he died after driving into the path of the lorry for no apparent reason ... There was no evidence of any prior defect on the car.' The verdict was accidental death.

In 1987 Sir Richard Body invited Mark to present a paper for the House of Commons Select Agriculture Committee about OP intoxication in farmers. The general public were also becoming interested in the topic and, following an appearance on the front page of *The Times,* Mark began receiving letters from across the country, all from people who claimed to be victims of chemical exposure.

He trawled through the medical literature and worked long into the night, without payment, to gather evidence, listening endlessly to stories of OP poisoning. I remember his study area at the time being a very cramped corridor in the family caravan. He got hold of research papers through inter-library loan, which for the fee of a pound enabled you to order up any technical paper and book through your local library. Most of his own heavy medical textbooks, which I found on his drooping shelves, bore an Oxfam stamp. He says:

> I found scientific journals dating back to the twenties, which showed exactly the same symptoms. But what interested me was that the symptoms these people described were frequently identical. They would include severe chronic fatigue, problems of coordination, sweating, dizziness, irritable bowel, breathlessness, eye problems, muscle twitching, tingling sensations, cramps, problems of temperature regulation, and various forms of mild paralysis. But all this is a consistent clinical pattern of damage to a variety of enzymes, such as cholinesterase in the nerves as well as other subtle affects. These patients had nearly all been told by doctors that they were neurotic malingerers, or were imagining their symptoms.

This interests me because I have suffered with CFS for 18 years and have done much research into my own case and into CFS in general. Of course the standard battery of tests which a GP gives to such a patient would not detect the kind of abnormalities that these patients have. It is imperative to do the right type of investigation to establish that these patients are genuinely ill, for example, there are many tests in which abnormalities are found in CFS — the hypothalamic pituitary adrenal axis, orthostatic hypotension, cytokine disregulation, ion channels, apoptosis, red cell morphology and oxygen transport.

Clearly most people today have some exposure to OPs and most do not end up with permanent illness. Most of the sufferers probably have a genetic predisposition, which involves polymorphisms in enzymes such as paraoxanase, which detoxify OPs. For example, many of the farmers who developed CFS after sheep dipping with the OP diazinon were later found to have such a polymorphism in PON1, the paraoxanase gene. There are also subtle forms of genetic inhibition whereby pesticides or other toxic compounds such as volatile organic compounds can, by adduction, become stuck to DNA causing the abnormal manufacture of some proteins. Epigenetics is another field of research, which has shown how OPs and other toxic molecules can also adversely affect protein production. The effects of this latter type of damage can be inherited. The neurologist Professor Peter Behan, of Glasgow University, has established that there is an association between OP exposure and a syndrome that is virtually indistinguishable from CFS.

The relevant point here may be the immuno-toxicity of OP pesticides. If OPs damage the immune system, victims would be more susceptible to infection. A high proportion of these fatigued patients develops a long-term illness after a viral infection by Epstein-Barr or Parvo B19, for example, rather than an obvious exposure to chemicals. But this begs the question has low-level chemical damage to the immune system paved the way for the continued inappropriate up-regulation of toxic immune proteins (cytokines), which could produce the long-term symptoms of CFS and which are normally only active whilst the virus is present.

In compiling his report, Mark had been struck by one observation: 'Some of the victims, especially those suffering long-term or occupational exposure, developed diseases that were close, if not identical to, the common form of motor neurone disease (MND).' He wondered whether there was a link between OP pesticides and what appeared to be the increasingly common occurrence of neurodegenerative diseases like MND, Parkinson's, Alzheimer's, multiple sclerosis (MS) and CFS. There is growing support for aspects of Mark's thesis. According to a paper published in the *Canadian Journal of Neurological Sciences* in 1987, researchers discovered 'that a significant correlation exists between pesticide use and the prevalence of Parkinson's disease.' These findings were buttressed by a 1993 paper in the US journal *Neurology*, which found 'evidence on behalf of an association between pesticide exposure, most prominently to insecticide products, and Parkinson's disease.' More recent studies have now also found that many Parkinson's sufferers carry one of the paraoxanase and/or cytochrome P450 polymorphisms, making them more at risk because they are slower at breaking down OP pesticides.

Mark believed that OPs also cause a loss of receptors in areas of the brain. This results in an increased uptake of calcium into nerve cells, which in turn causes a ballooning effect attributable to a vacuolation of neurones in the brainstem. Neuronal vacuoles have been noted in BSE post-mortems, and a paper co-authored by Professor J.B. Cavanagh, formerly of the MRC, described such vacuoles as being 'apparently limited to organophosphorous neuropathy'. In white blood cells a high calcium influx is also found and is associated with excessive programmed cell death or apoptosis. Interestingly, when I had these tests done my white cells were found to have very high calcium levels and apoptosis 45–50% above the norm. The widespread use of pesticides has accelerated far ahead of any objective scientific evaluation of them. 'There was a World Health Organization report in 1981 saying we don't know what the long-term, low-level effects of pesticides are — we should find out.'

After Mark made the 1988 *Open Space* TV documentary *Aggrochemicals* about OPs and human health, the poet Ted Hughes wrote to him with 'a million congratulations — Purdey's argument was clear, self-evident, inexorable. So simple. One bull's-eye after another. You've planted a big bomb. They can't hide from the camera, can they? They're as scared as we are.'

All this was controversial and didn't win Mark any friends either in the pesticides industry or certain sectors of government. What followed was to test both him and his family to breaking point.

In the late eighties Mark bought some land near Crediton at an auction. A man who during the next year almost destroyed Mark and his family bought the adjacent farmhouse at the same sale.

He'd been very pally with us before we moved in, but his dress, his demeanour, even his way of talking, all struck me as odd. Then he moved in, and began making our lives hell. He'd argue about everything. He initiated problems with the electricity cables running across his land. I learned he'd been telephoning the water board five days a week, trying to get us cut off. He had eight Doberman dogs that were chasing our cows. Some nights we couldn't sleep, wondering what was going to happen next. He had an array of serious guns and fired a Kalashnikov over our property and into the milking parlour on several occasions and let off detonations when the milk lorry arrived. At first I thought he was just a nutter, but over the months things escalated, I reported the incidents to the police and I revised my opinion.

One day when Mark was due to go to address a House of Commons select committee, he found himself barricaded in by one of his neighbour's war memorabilia vehicles. 'It was parked across the front of the driveway. We couldn't get the lorry in to pick up the milk and I couldn't get out and missed the crucial meeting. I don't believe that this was a coincidence because the blockage occurred at the precise time that I needed to get out.'

On another occasion, which Mark calls 'Bloody Sunday', their neighbour began firing at their milking parlour while Mark sheltered inside. Margaret, who was nine months pregnant, called the police, who said Mark would have to be shot before they could do anything.

He riddled the base of our milking parlour with shots and told the police that he'd been shooting vermin. The policeman who came out on that occasion was very friendly and said, 'We know who this man is. You realize people are employed to behave in this way. I can't give you any more clues, but you were the one who took the pesticide case to court, weren't you?'

It was a clever campaign because it was one of sustained intimidation. He never actually harmed us and he was always quite civil, if a little eccentric, to us face to face. The campaign 'worked' and things got so bad that we decided to sell up and buy a farm near Haverfordwest in Dyfed.

The night before the family was due to move in, as the *Guardian* reported on 2 June 1988, it was burned to the ground. 'The local police said it was an electrical fault, but no electricity was switched on at the time.' They went into hiding. Mark points out that in the US it is well known that campaigners like him are subjected to harassment and attempts to discredit them, so why not here? 'The week after we left, our former neighbour put his house on the market and moved on.' Another incident occurred on 28 December 1991 while the family was away for Christmas. A small section of their barn wall, which they hadn't been working on, 'fell down'. The part that happened to fall was adjacent to a caravan, which contained Marks's medical library and his papers. The wall crushed most of the caravan. The height to width ratio of the stone wall – 2 foot thick to about 11 foot high – makes it highly unlikely that the wall would just blow over. 'We had just got planning permission to convert the barn, and the wall had stood for about 200 years. It's true the footings were not brilliant, but taken together the timing of the fall, during the few days in a year we were all away, seems too much of a coincidence. We were sure the phones were tapped at that time and it was easy to plan such an operation.' The newspaper picture shows Mark holding aloft his saxophone, which was salvaged from the wreckage, playing it to his cows.

Over the next few years, alarming incidents occurred with increasing regularity. In the spring of 1993, one of Mark's calves was born with BSE to a cow with BSE. The night before a news story about this was due to appear in the *Independent*, the steel cable which carried his telephone line was found cut and this was confirmed as a deliberate act by the police. It was impossible for the media to contact Mark. What are the chances of an aimless hoodlum coming to this isolated spot, coming onto his land, climbing up a telegraph pole and cutting the steel cable and line for the sheer hell of it? It had to have been a 'job' connected with the news story and his campaign.

Another incident occurred when he was in the process of starting up an organic milk service with Express Dairies when, one Christmas Eve, a MAFF inspector turned up and suddenly claimed his milk, which had hitherto been in the premium 'Band A' for hygiene, was tainted. By what, wasn't specified, but the inspector said he thought he could detect a whiff of apples. Mark had no apple trees on his farm and had never fed apples to his cows. No test is made at the inspection – it is totally subjective. Because of the holiday period, he was unable to get an independent assessment of the milk's quality or to get any legal advice. By the time this had been obtained, Express Dairies had not surprisingly cancelled the order and a year's hard preparatory work went down the pan.

On the Saturday that the Press Association put out a news release about his meeting with MAFF officials, his phone went dead. Mark says all this left him 'financially and emotionally derelict'.

In the spring of 1996 it was announced that BSE had infected humans in the form of variant CJD, and several leading scientists – all specialists in spongiform brain diseases – met with tragic deaths.

Dr Clive Bruton, curator of the Corsellis Collection Brain Bank at Runwell Hospital in Essex, was found dead in his crashed car after a heart attack. He had been publicly arguing that deaths from CJD were going unrecognized because it was assumed that Alzheimer's disease, which has similar symptoms, was the cause.

The MP Teresa Gorman, who had successfully campaigned to stop the Corsellis Collection from being dispersed, said this was a uniquely valuable resource in that it contained the brains of people who died of sporadic CJD before BSE appeared. Comparison with CJD victims might show that the same brain plaques were in evidence before BSE – or perhaps not. 'This should have been examined in the context of BSE,' she said. 'I do think Mark Purdey's theory deserves more attention, but there's a huge vested interest at the SEAC end, with a lot of members from industry on this committee. They have a position to maintain and it has been difficult to get funding for alternative research.'

Unusual incidents seemed to go hand in hand with spongiform encephalopathy research. In the spring of 1996 the Nobel Prize-winner Dr Carleton Gajdusek, renowned for his research into kuru, a variant of CJD, which occurs in New Guinea tribespeople, was arrested in America for sex offences. According to the National Institute of Health where Gajdusek worked in Bethesda, Maryland, his journals, detailing traditional practices in the tribes he worked with, had been in the public domain for 30 years. The *Observer* of 16 February 1997 reported: 'On 4 April 1996 as Dr Gajdusek was flying back from a conference on BSE in Geneva, FBI agents were raiding both his office and his home in Maryland. They took away his files, disks, photographs, film and notebooks. The same evening when he drew into his driveway with a colleague, a dozen FBI agents leapt from cover and arrested the 72-year-old at gunpoint.' Gajdusek protested his innocence but went to prison.

In April 1998, on the eve of Mark's day-long hearing at the BSE Inquiry, the Government announced they would aid research into his BSE theory. This point received wide coverage in the press, but as time went on it became clear that this had been a PR exercise all along.

'They have failed to grant funding to any proposals to date, including my own, and so the research still hasn't happened. The upshot of this is that the public has stopped funding my research because they think the Government is now paying for it – and I have been left high and dry.'

The arrival in 1998 of the Data Protection Act enabled Mark, on payment of 50p a time, to make applications to various organizations to disclose their documentation in which he was named. Mark relates:

An application to the UK Government Departments for my personal data revealed much of what had been going on behind the scenes. Repeated requests by Environment Minister, Michael Meacher, to personally meet with me had been deliberately stymied by his own officials. The Minister eventually broke through the barrage of officials to make direct arrangements with me for the meeting but it was postponed on five separate occasions, and when it finally took place it was taken over by the official and I got nowhere. Other documents revealed how the British Agrochemical Association had been organizing a 'joint initiative' with the Ministry of Agriculture's own grant funding department to channel public funds into a live animal trial that had been deliberately designed to refute my theory. Since the BSE Inquiry had largely rejected the official scrapie-BSE hypothesis and found in favour of some aspects of my hypothesis, the UK Government responded by setting up a further mini-Inquiry to re-look at the origins of BSE. The resulting publication, known as the 'Gabriel Horne Report', employed judicious sleight of word and bogus information to discredit my theory, either through the incompetence of the authors or through deliberate obfuscation.

There were eight main points (see the 'Warble Fly in the Ointment' chapter) that Mark disputed, but perhaps the biggest blunder was that Horne stated that the use of OP warblecides had ceased in the UK by 1982. If true, this would knock out the OP relevance, because BSE really took off much later in the late eighties and early nineties, and in fact 1982 was the year the Act was introduced and the treatment started.

'When I attempted to sue the Government for defamation and loss of income resulting from this report, which was circulated in a global publication, they pleaded "qualified privilege" of the expert committee. They then spun out the legal communications beyond the one year after the publication date, thereby exempting themselves from my claim.' 'Political' science like this is a manifest nonsense and fortunately for its proponents the major errors in Horne escaped the radar of our science journalists, who continue to espouse its 'expert' findings to this day.

After the broadcasting of the BBC2 Correspondent film *Mad Cows and An Englishman* which featured Mark's investigations into TSEs, the Government tried to appease the mounting public interest by inviting him to resubmit an application to them for funding.

After sitting on my application for a year and a half, they focused on the most fastidious, nit-picking comments in the peer-review appraisal, inflating them to the level of serious science and then using this as a basis for their rejection. Ironically, immediately after this episode the author of the most irrational and irrelevant critique was promoted to the Government's 'TSE surveillance steering committee' – presumably as a reward for his good work.

But as time went on Mark started to gain support from many quarters. Global media coverage focused on both the 'personal struggle' and 'scientific perspectives' of his story. His work was published in peer-reviewed journals and in news and feature articles in UK newspapers, and was also presented in radio and TV documentary programmes over the years, some being broadcast around the world. Many of his films achieved top viewer ratings for the series, with excellent feedback, including national newspaper preview and review features. His work gained a large following, across a wide cross section of people, such as many high ranking scientists with whom he collaborated, Government Ministers and finally HRH Prince Charles, who invited him, together with Dr David Brown, to a personal meeting at Highgrove. His article summarizing his research, called 'Educating Rida', was highly commended and was a runner-up in the Martha Gellhorn investigative journalism award of 2003.

Invitations came in to give lectures and presentations at a number of prestigious institutions – the Spongiform Encephalopathy Advisory Committee (SEAC), the Medical Research Council, the Edinburgh International Science Festival, the Prion Diseases and Copper Conference at Cambridge University, the Italian centre for TSE surveillance at Torino University Hospital, the Harvard Medical School and the US Environmental Protection Agency.

But Mark consistently found some humbler doors closer to home resolutely closed to him. He used to say, 'It's a piece of cake to get long articles published in peer-reviewed journals, compared to getting a short piece about me published in the *Independent* or the *Telegraph*. It's ironic that I'm considered "OK" to lecture at Harvard and give presentations to the EPA, SEAC and the MRC, but not good enough for the likes of UK hacks Steve Connor and Roger Highfield, who seek to muzzle me at all costs.'

Some of the most intense opposition to Mark's work came from a West Country pesticide campaigner.

It was uncanny, she seemed to know virtually everything I was doing and what I was writing – she thought I was dangerous. On one occasion she seemed quite mysteriously to get hold of a synopsis of an article which had been sent to a peer-reviewer. She didn't want it to be published. I was bemused, because apart from this being unethical it was none of her business. She was not qualified to peer-review and I don't think she had ever published anything in a peer-reviewed journal or written anything of interest. On another occasion when one of my TV films was about to be broadcast she spent most of the day on the phone to anyone connected with the film at Channel 4, trying to get the broadcast stopped. She couldn't have seen the film, or even a synopsis of it, and yet she clearly wanted it pulled at all costs, because she thought it was dangerous in some way. In the end, thankfully, it was broadcast and as far as I know no one suffered as a result of what was said in the film.

Another problem that Mark came up against was in getting right of reply. An example of this was a long article in the *Daily Telegraph* written by Sir Aaron Klug, then President of the Royal Society, in which he sought to quash what he saw as a media myth, that OPs caused BSE. Although Mark was not mentioned by name, it is clear that he was in the frame and Mark submitted some counter-arguments to the article. 'The science editor, Dr Roger Highfield, told me that when you make scientific assertions you have to reference them (as if this was beyond me) so I sent him a page of references. (Had Sir Aaron Klug done this?) Highfield then said the piece was too long and I would have to cut it right down. I cut it right down and then he said I hadn't dealt with all of Sir Aaron Klug's points and he wouldn't publish any of it.'

On another occasion a leading sketch writer on the *Independent*, Simon Carr, had written a piece about Mark's work for his paper, but the article was instantly dismissed when submitted to the science editor, Steve Connor, as soon as Mark's name came up.

I'll leave the last word to Mark's MP at this time, (now Lord) Tom King, who was a public supporter. 'Purdey is a very remarkable man,' says King, 'an individual farmer who didn't believe the official statements on BSE and who had painstakingly pursued a theory which is a classic piece of scientific investigation and intelligent observation of his own cattle. My wife is a farmer and I have dipped sheep with OPs: the sheep passed out and we thought they were dead. These compounds were launched without adequate warnings.'

Table 1

Key TSE Clusters Around the World

Their correlation with locations where munitions have been manufactured, tested, stored, incinerated or dumped

USA				
Location	Date	TSE type	Munitions connection	Sonic source
Tucson, AZ	1978	CJD cluster	Missile factory workers	Workshop tests
Fort Collins, CO	1968	CWD cluster in wild/ captive deer	Missile silos, Rocky Flats nuclear munitions factory leak, munition incineration in Lyons cement kiln and 11 million gal of nerve agent at Rocky Mountain Arsenal	Quarry explosions, rifle shooting, LF jets, Front Range tectonic fault line
Mt Horeb, WI	2000	CWD cluster in wild deer	Clean-up/incineration of munitions at Badger ammunition plant in 1999, Hercules flight path	Explosions for new road, rifle shooting, quake epicentre, LF jets
Kimball, NE	2000	CWD cluster in wild deer	Incineration of Badger munitions at Kimball incinerator in 1999, missile silos	LF jets, rifle shooting
White Sands Missile Range, NM	2000	CWD cluster in wild deer	Missile and bomb testing range	Missile explosions
Mission, TX	1960s	Scrapie cluster	Former military air base (World War II), bomb storage	Under former takeoff flight path
Garden State, NJ	1990s	CJD cluster	Fort Dix military camp, MacGuire air base	LF jets, gun and shell explosions

Location	Date	TSE type	Munitions connection	Sonic source
Mabton, WA	2004	1st US BSE	Hanford nuclear weapons plant, Yakima military training camp, Othello air base	LF jets, shell explosions
Spokane, WA	2004	1st US vCJD	Hanford nuclear weapons plant, Yakima military training camp, Othello air base	LF jets, shell explosions
CANADA				
Location	Date	TSE type	Munitions connection	Sonic source
Nameo, AL	2001	1st Canadian CWD captive deer	Nameo military air base	Under takeoff flight path
Leduc, AL	2003	1st US BSE cow reared here	Leduc International Airport (mainly civilian)	Under takeoff flight path
Tulliby Lake, AL	2003	1st Canadian BSE	Cold Lake air base and air weapons/cruise missile test range	Under LF jet practise circuit/ Hercules flight path
Hillmond, SA	2002	CWD cluster in farmed elk	Fallout from Cold Lake air weapons test range	Under Lloydminster Airport takeoff path/Hercules flight path. Gas well pumping
Manitou, SA	2002	CWD cluster in wild deer	Camp Wainwright tank shelling range, detonation/incineration of waste munitions, chemical munitions	Tank shelling, Manitou rifle shooting range
Between Lloydminster and Saskatoon, SA	2002	1st vCJD	Fallout from Camp Wainwright/Cold Lake air weapons range	LF jets, munition explosions

(Cont.)

UK				
Location	Date	TSE type	Munitions connection	Sonic source
Burnham-on-Sea, Somerset	2000	vCJD cases	Puriton ordnance factory, former World War II air base	LF military jets
Armthorpe, near Doncaster	2000	vCJD cluster	RAF Finningley	LF military jets flight path, Concorde visits
Queniborough, Leicestershire	1996	vCJD cluster	Queniborough ordnance depot, World War II bomber crash Mountsorrel quarry	LF military jets, Kegworth International Airport flight path, Concorde visits
Villages north of Tenby, South Wales	2000	vCJD cluster	Castlemartin and Pendine Sands tank shelling/bomb test ranges	LF military jets
South-west Lancashire	1999	vCJD cases	Chorley ordnance factory/munition incinerator	LF military jets
Sunderland area	1998	vCJD cases	Cokeworks munition incinerator	
Lympstone, Devon	2000	vCJD cases	Lympstone marine camp	LF aircraft flight path (Exeter Airport), Concorde visits
Eastleigh, Southampton	1998	vCJD cases	Eastleigh works munition factory	LF aircraft flight path (Southampton Airport)
East Chinnock/ Stoke, Somerset	1992	sCJD cluster	Yeovilton naval air base	LF military jets

Location	Date	TSE type	Munitions connection	Sonic source
Villages west of Ashford, Kent	1996	vCJD cluster	Local woodlands used as chemical/ conventional bomb depots in World War II, Smarden insecticide factory, World War II bomber/USAF air bases at Headcorn/High Halden, World War II 'Bomb Alley'	LF military jets, flight paths into Heathrow Airport and local Headcorn Airport]
Villages north of Woodbridge, Suffolk	1975	vCJD cluster	Orfordness nuclear/ conventional bomb factories, bomber air base and crash landing in Parham village	LF military jet flight path
Weston Longeville	1998	vCJD case	West Longeville US bomber base/bomber crash site World War II munition stores	LF military jets
FAR EAST				
Location	**Date**	**TSE type**	**Munitions connection**	**Sonic source**
Guam	2002	CJD case	World War II chemical munitions buried in victim's land	LF military jets, tropical storms, earthquake tectonic fault lines
Highlands of New Guinea	1950s	Kuru cluster	World War II US bomber crashes/ exploding bombs	Bomb explosions, thunderstorm belt, earthquake tectonic fault line
Obhiro, Hokkaido, Japan	1950s	Scrapie cluster	World War II army weapons test range	LF military jets
Fuji valley, Japan	1950s	S/familial CJD cluster	Munitions/film factories, aluminium alloy factories	Volcanic/ earthquake belt

(Cont.)

ITALY				
Location	Date	TSE type	Munitions connection	Sonic source
Parma region, Italy	1975	sCJD cluster	Munitions factory	
Ragusa, Sicily	2000	BSE cases	Comiso USAF air base. Nuclear cruise missile base	LF jet flight path
Trapani, Sicily	1998	BSE cases	Trapani Bergi NATO air base	LF jet/Stealth jet flight path
Menfi, Sicily	2001	vCJD case	Sciacca World War II bomber air base, intense bombing	LF jets/quarry explosions
Aspromonte, Calabria	1990	S/familial CJD clusters	Ordnance/nuclear waste dumping, explosions	LF jets, explosions, earthquake tectonic fault line
Barbagia Monte, Sardinia	1995	Scrapie clusters	Ordnance/toxic waste dumping	LF jets, quarry explosions
Assemini, Sardinia	1999	Scrapie cluster	Decimmannu NATO air base	LF military and civilian jet flight paths
Arborea, Sardinia	2001	1st BSE case	Capo de Frasco air weapons test range	LF jet practice circuit/explosions

Table 2

Key Clusters of Human TSEs Around the World

Their correlation with sources of piezoelectric siliaceous microcrystal pollutants

Location of vCJD clusters	Year	Local source of silicate piezoelectric microcrystals	Local source of sonic shocks
Adswood	2000	Brick and tile factory	Manchester Airport flight path
Armthorpe	2000	Brick crushing works, former 'Gunhills' range	RAF Finningley flight path
Queniborough	1996	Former chemical munitions/detonator factory, dyeworks, gypsum factory, USAF World War II bomber crashes, Mountsorrel quarry	Low-fly jet practice route, Concorde visits to airshow
Eastleigh	1998	Local brick works	Southampton Airport flight path
Villages north of Tenby	2000	Potteries. Pendine Sands/Penally/Castlemartin/Pembrey/Manorbier weapons test ranges	Low-fly jet practice route, tank/bomb/shooting ranges
Burnham-on-Sea	2000	Puriton ordnance factory, Weston naval bomb test range, World War II airbase	Low-fly jet practice route
Lympstone	2000	Lympstone Marine Camp, Woodbury Common practice range, barium/manganese silicates in estuary cliff	Exeter Airport flight path, former Concorde visits

(Cont.)

Ashford villages	1990s	Brick/tile factories, munitions stored in woods, USAF World War II bomber crashes, World War II 'Bomb Alley', Lydd firing range	Low-fly jet practice route, Heathrow flight path, Lydd/Hythe firing ranges
Glasgow suburbs	2000	Bishopton ordnance factory	Glasgow International Airport flight paths
Sunderland	1998	Cokeworks munition incinerator, glassworks	
Essex	1970	Shoeburyness minition incinerator/firing range/sea dumping	Shoeburyness firing range/Stansted Airport flight path
South Somerset	1992	Yeovilton naval air base	Low-fly naval jets
Orava, Slovakia	1960s	Ferrosilicate steel factories	
Poltar, Slovakia	1960s	Glass factories	
Calabria, Italy Parma, Italy	1990s	Munitions/steel factories	Explosions
Papua New Guinea	1950s	Crashed USAF/Japanese World War II bombers	Earthquake zone tectonic sonic shocks, exploding bombs
Fuji, Japan	1990s	Munition, ferrosilicate alloy, film, dye factories, Fuji volcano	Volcanic tectonic shocks
Tucson, Arizona	1980s	Missile factory	Missile testing

Principal Sources and Further Reading

Chapter 1 A Warble Fly in the Ointment

Bouldin, T.W., and Cavanagh, J.B., 'Organophosphorous neuropathy, I. A teased-fiber study of the spatio-temporal spread of axonol degeneration', *Am. J. Path.* 1979, 94, 241–52

Bouldin, T.W., and Cavanagh, J.B., 'Organophosphorous neuropathy, II. A fine-structural study of the early stages of axonal degeneration', *Am. J. Path.*, 1979, 94, 253–70

Bounias, M., and Purdey, M., 'Transmissible spongiform encephalopathies: a family of etiologically complex diseases – a review', *Sci. Total Environ.*, 2002 Oct 7, 297 (1–3), 1–19. Review

Brown, D., Hafiz, F., Glassmith, L., et al., 'Consequences of manganese replacement of copper for prion protein function and proteinase resistance', *EMBO J.* 2000, 19 (6), 1180–6

Bush, A.I., 'Metals and neuroscience. Current opinion', *Chem. Biol.* 2000 Apr., 4 (2), 184–91. Review

Deloncle, R., et al., 'Free radical generation of protease-resistant prion after substitution of manganese for copper in bovine brain homogenate', *Neurotoxicology* 2006 May, 27 (3), 437–44. Epub 14 Feb. 2006

Gordon, I., Abdulla, E.M., Campbell, I.C., and Whatley, S.A., 'Phosmet induces up-regulation of surface levels of cellular prion protein', *Neuroreport* 1998, 9 (7), 1391–5

Hesketh, S., Sassoon, J., Knight, R., Hopkins, J., and Brown, D.R., 'Elevated manganese levels in blood and central nervous system occur before onset of clinical signs in scrapie and bovine spongiform encephalopathy', *J. Anim. Sci.* 2007 June, 86 (6), 1596–609. Epub Feb. 12 2007

Kim, N.H., et al., 'Effect of transition metals (Mn, Cu, Fe) and deoxycholic acid (DA) on the conversion of PrPC to PrPres', *FASEB J.* 2005 May, 19 (7), 783–5. Epub 9 Mar. 2005

Kimberlin, R.H., Millson, G.C., Bountiff, L., and Collis, S.C., 'A comparison of the biochemical changes induced in mouse brain cuprizone toxicity and by scrapie infection', *J. Comp Pathol.* 1974 Apr., 84 (2), 263–70

Pattison, I.H., Clarke, M.C., Haig, D.A., and Jebbett, J.N., 'Cell cultures from mice affected with scrapie or fed with cuprizone', *Res. Vet. Sci.* 1971 Sept., 12 (5),

478–80. No abstract available

Purdey, M., 'Mad Cows and Warble Flies', *Ecologist* 1994, 24 (3), 100–4

Purdey, M., 'Are organophosphate pesticides involved in the causation of BSE? Hypothesis based on a literature review and limited trials on BSE cattle', *J. of Nutritional Medicine* 1994, 4 (1), 43–82

Purdey, M., 'The UK epidemic of BSE: slow virus or chronic pesticide-initiated modification of the prion protein? Part 1: Mechanisms for a chemically induced pathogenesis/transmissibility', *Medical Hypotheses* 1996 May, 46 (5), 429–43

Purdey, M., 'The UK epidemic of BSE: slow virus or chronic pesticide-initiated modification of the prion protein? Part 2: An epidemiological perspective', *Med. Hypotheses* 1996 May, 46 (5), 445–54

Purdey, M., 'High-dose exposure to systemic phosmet insecticide modifies the phosphatidylinositol anchor on the prion protein: the origins of new variant transmissible spongiform encephalopathies?' *Med. Hypotheses* 1998 Feb., 50 (2), 91–111. Review

Purdey, M., 'Ecosystems supporting clusters of sporadic TSEs demonstrate excesses of the radical-generating divalent cation, manganese, and deficiencies of antioxidant co-factors Cu, Se, Fe, Zn. Does a foreign cation substitution at prion protein's Cu domain initiate TSE?' *Med. Hypotheses* 2000, 54 (2), 278–306

Purdey, M., 'The Mn loaded/Cu depleted bovine brain fails to neutralize incoming shock bursts of low frequency infrasound; the origins of BSE?' *Cattle Practice* 2002 Oct., 10 (4), 311–25

Wong, B.S., Chen, S.G., Colucci, M., Xie, Z., Pan, T., Liu, T., Sy, M.S., Gambetti, P., and Brown, D.R., 'Aberrant metal binding by prion protein in human prion disease', *J. Neurochem.* 2001, 78, 1400–8

Chapter 2 The Crystal Grail

D'Alessandro, M., et al., 'High incidence of Creutzfeldt-Jakob disease in rural Calabria, Italy', *Lancet* 1998 Dec. 19–26, 352 (9145), 1989–90

Hay, I., *R.O.F.: The Story of the Royal Ordnance Factories 1939–1948*, HMSO, London 1948

Matthews, W.B., 'Epidemiology of Creutzfeldt-Jakob disease in England and Wales', *J. Neurol. Neurosurg. Psychiatry* 1975 Mar., 38 (3), 210–13

Parry, A., et al., 'Long term survival in a patient with variant Creutzfeldt-Jakob disease treated with intraventricular pentosan polysulphate', *J. Neurol. Neurosurg. Psychiatry* 2007 Feb. 21. [Epub ahead of print]

Purdey, M., 'Elevated levels of ferrimagnetic metals in foodchains supporting the Guam cluster of neurodegeneration: do metal nucleated crystal contaminants [corrected] evoke magnetic fields that initiate the progressive pathogenesis of neurodegeneration?' *Med. Hypotheses* 2004, 63 (5), 793–809. Erratum in: *Med. Hypotheses* 2005, 65 (6), 1207

Wientjens, D.P., et al., 'Risk factors for Creutzfeldt-Jakob disease: a reanalysis of case-control studies', *Neurology* 1996 May, 46 (5), 1287–91. Review

Zanusso, G., et al., 'Simultaneous occurrence of spongiform encephalopathy in a man and his cat in Italy', *Lancet* 1998 Oct. 3, 352 (9134), 1116–7

Chapter 3 Sheep May Safely Graze

Agrimi, U., et al., 'Epidemic of transmissible spongiform encephalopathy in sheep and goats in Italy', *Lancet* 1999 Feb. 13, 353 (9152), 560–1. No abstract available

D'Alessandro, M., et al., 'High incidence of Creutzfeldt-Jakob disease in rural Calabria, Italy', *Lancet* 1998 Dec. 19–26, 352 (9145), 1989–90

Kim, N.H., et al., 'Effect of transition metals (Mn, Cu, Fe) and deoxycholic acid (DA) on the conversion of PrPC to PrPres', *FASEB J.* 2005 May, 19 (7), 783–5. Epub 9 Mar. 2005

Mitrova, E., 'Some new aspects of CJD epidemiology in Slovakia', *Eur. J. Epidemiol.* 1991 Sept., 7 (5), 439–49

Mitrova, E., and Bronis, M., ' "Clusters" of CJD in Slovakia: the first statistically significant temporo-spatial accumulations of rural cases', *Eur. J. Epidemiol.* 1991 Sept., 7 (5), 450–6

Mitrova, E., Huncaga, S., Hocman, G., Nyitrayova, O., and Tatara, M., ' "Clusters" of CJD in Slovakia: the first laboratory evidence of scrapie', *Eur. J. Epidemiol.* 1991 Sept., 7 (5), 520–3. Review

Palsson, P.A., *Rida in Iceland and its Epidemiology. Slow transmissible diseases of the nervous system*, Vol. 1, Academic Press London 1979

Purdey, M., 'Ecosystems supporting clusters of sporadic TSEs demonstrate excesses of the radical-generating divalent cation manganese and deficiencies of antioxidant co-factors Cu, Se, Fe, Zn. Does a foreign cation substitution at prion protein's Cu domain initiate TSE?' *Med. Hypotheses* 2000 Feb., 54 (2), 278–306. Review

Chapter 4 Becquerels on the Brain

Bara, M., Guiet-Bara, A., and Durlach, J., 'Regulation of sodium and potassium pathways by magnesium in cell membranes', *Magnesium Res.* 1993, 6 (2), 167–77

Briscoe, C.L.S., *Blue Ribbon Panel Committee Action Report on Radioactive Contamination in Guam Between 1946–1958*, ed. Castro, W.M. From the offices of Senator Angel L.G. Santos and Senator Mark Forbes, Agana, Guam, 12 November 2002

Calne, D.B., Eisen, A., McGeer, E., and Spencer, P., 'Alzheimer's disease, Parkinson's disease and motor neurone disease: a biotrophic interaction between ageing and environment. A hypothesis', *Lancet* 1986 Nov. 8, 1067–70

Celestial, Robert N., and Perez, W.C., 'Radiation Fall Out Guam'

Cutler, R.G., Pederson, W.A., Camandola, S., Rothskin, J.D., and Mattson, M.P., 'Evidence that accumulation of ceramides and cholesterol esters mediate oxidative stress induced death of motor neurones in ALS', *Annals of Neurol.* 2002, 52

Da Silva, F.J.J.R., and Williams, R.J.P., *The Biological Chemistry of the Elements*, 2nd edn, Oxford University Press, Oxford 2001

Donaldson, L.R., Seymour, A.H., and Nevissi, A.E., 'University of Washington's radioecological studies in the Marshall Islands, 1946–1977', *Health Physics* 1997 July, 73 (1), 214–22

Eisenbud, M., and Gesell, T., *Environmental Radioactivity*, 4th edn, Academic Press, London 1997

Fowler, S., 'Plant toxin linked to Guam dementia', *New Scientist* 1987 August 3, 31

Gajdusek, D.C., 'Foci of motor neurone disease in high incidence in isolated populations of East Asia and the Western Pacific', in Rowland, L.P. (ed.), *Human Motor Neurone Disease*, Raven Press, New York 1982, pp. 363–93

Gajdusek, D.C., 'Hypothesis: interference with axonal transport of neurofilament as a common pathogenetic mechanism in certain diseases of the CNS', *New England J. Med.* 1985, 312 (11), 714–18

Halliwell, B., and Gutteridge, J.M.C. (eds), *Free Radicals in Biology and Medicine*, 2nd edn, Clarendon Press, Oxford 1989

Kan, M., Wang, F., To, B., Gabriel, J.L., and McKeehan, W.L., 'Divalent cations and heparin/heparan sulphate cooperate to control assembly and activity of the fibroblast growth factor receptor complex', *J. Biol. Chem.* 1996, 271 (42), 26143–8

Miller, W.R., and Sanzolone, R.F., *Investigation of the Possible Connection of Rock and Soil Geochemistry to the Occurrence of High Rates of Neurodegenerative*

Diseases on Guam and a Hypothesis for the Cause of the Diseases. Open-File Report 02-475. US Dept. of the Interior, US Geological Survey, Denver, CO 80225, 2002

'Operation Crossroads' DNA6032F, United States atmospheric nuclear weapons tests. Nuclear test personnel review, 1946

Perl, D.P., 'ALS-Parkinsonism-dementia complex of Guam', in Esire, M.M., and Morris, J.H. (eds), *Neuropathology of Dementia*, Cambridge University Press, Cambridge 1997, pp. 268–92

Purdey, M., 'BSE: Are we being fed a lie?' *Ecologist* 2002, 32 (9), 33–7

Purdey, M., 'Does an infrasonic acoustic shock wave resonance of the manganese 3+ loaded/copper depleted prion protein initiate the pathogenesis of TSE?' *Med. Hypotheses* 2003, 60 (6), 797–820

Purdey, M., 'Chronic barium intoxication disrupts sulphated proteoglycan synthesis: a hypothesis for the origins of multiple sclerosis', *Med. Hypotheses* 2004, 62 (5), 746–54

Purdey, M., 'Elevated levels of ferrimagnetic metals in food chains supporting the Guam cluster of neurodegeneration: do metal nucleated crystal contaminants evoke magnetic fields that initiate the progressive pathogenesis of neurodegeneration?' *Med. Hypotheses* 2004, 63 (5), 793–809. Erratum in *Med. Hypotheses* 2005, 65 (6), 1207

Sacks, O., *The Island of the Colour-blind and Cycad Island*, Alfred Knopf, New York 1997

Sanderson, Vancil I., sworn statement, Tori Kae Nigro, Notary Public, State of Nevada. Recorded in Washoe County. No. 99-37452-2, 30 August 2001

Schwarcz, R., and Meldrum, B., 'Excitatory amino acid antagonists provide a therapeutic approach to neurological disorders', *Lancet* 1985 July 20, 140–3

Siddique, T., et al., *Nature Genetics* 2001 October 3

Spencer, P.S., and Schaumburg, H.H. (eds), *Experimental and Clinical Neurotoxicology*, 2nd edn, Oxford University Press, New York 2000

WHO, Geneva 1990: *Barium*, Environmental Health Criteria 107, international programme on chemical safety

Chapter 5 To the Ends of the Earth

Aschner, M., and Aschner, J.L., 'Manganese neurotoxicity: cellular effects and blood-brain barrier transport', *Neurosci. Biobehavioural Rev.* 1990, 15, 333–40

Burt, T., 'Public health issues in east Arnhem Land, Northern Territory: Progress Report, Public Health Research, Angurugu Community 1990–1992', Menzies School of Health Research, Darwin 1992, pp. 1–12

Burt, T., et al., 'Machado-Joseph disease in east Arnhem Land, Australia: chromosome 14q32.1 expanded repeat confirmed in four families', *Neurology* 1996 Apr., 46 (4), 1118–22

Cawte, J., and Florence, M., 'Environmental source of manganese on Groote Eylandt, North Australia', *Lancet* 1987, ii, 1484

Cawte, J., and Florence, M., 'A manganic milieu in North Australia: ecological manganism', *Int. J. Biosocial Res.* 1989, 11, 1–14

Cawte, J., Hams, G., and Kilburn, C., 'Manganism in a neurological ethnic complex in northern Australia', *Lancet* 1987 May 30, 1257

Cawte, J., and Kilburn, C., *Manganese and Metabolism; Groote Eylandt, Northern Territory Conference Proceedings*, University of Queensland Press, 1987

Findlay, A.W., 'Dust monitoring and dust control at the manganese mine, Groote Eylandt'. Report by senior lecturer in occupational hygiene, National Institute in Occupational Health and Safety, Building A27, University of Sydney, 17 October 1988, 1–43

Florence, T.M., Stauber, J.L., and Fardy, J.J., 'Ecological studies of manganese on Groote Eylandt', CSIRO Division of Energy Chemistry, Lucas Heights, NSW, Australia, 1988

Purdey, M., 'The pathogenesis of Machado-Joseph Disease: a high manganese/low magnesium initiated CAG expansion mutation in susceptible genotypes?' *J. Am. Coll. Nutr.* 2004 Dec., 23 (6), 714S–29S. Review

Spillett, P., 'Machado Joseph Disease. The probability of inheritance from the Portuguese via Makassan sailors to the Aborigines of Arnhem Land and Groote Eylandt', 1992, pp. 31–9. Commissioned report held at Northern Territory Museum of Arts and Sciences, Darwin

Chapter 6 The Wasting Lands

Alldredge, A.W., Lipscomb, J.F., and Whicker, F.W., 'Forage intake rates of mule deer estimated with fallout Cs-137', *J. Wildlife Management* 1974, 38, 508–15

Alldredge, A.W., Whicker, W.F., and Hakonson, T.E., 'Retention of intravenously administered Cs 134 in mule deer'; 10th annual progress report on AEC contract AT (11-1)-1156. Dept. Radiol. Radiat. Biol., Colorado State University, Fort Collins, 1972, p. 14–17

Arthur, W.J., '111 Plutonium intake by mule deer at Rocky Flats, Colorado'. MS thesis, Colorado State University, Fort Collins, 1977

Arthur, W.J., and Alldredge, A.W., 'Soil ingestion by mule deer in north central Colorado', *Journal of Range Management* 1979, 32 (1), 67–71

Brown, D., 'Prion and prejudice; normal protein and the synapse', *Trends in Neurosciences* 2001, 24 (2), 85–90

Crom, R., 'Cluster of CJD cases in Tucson'. Report, the Epidemic Intelligence Service of the Arizona Department of Health Services, Phoenix 1990

D'Alessandro, M., Petraroli, R., Ladogana, A., and Pocchiari, M., 'High incidence of CJD in rural Calabria', *Lancet* 1998, 352, 1989–90

Dougherty, J., 'EPA finds plutonium, dioxin in cement dust', *Concrete Facts* 1993, 2 (4) 1–4 (PO Box 58, Laporte, CO 80535)

Hakonson, T.E., 'Tissue distribution and excretion of Cs 134 in the mule deer'. MS thesis, Colorado State University, Fort Collins, 1967

Hakonson, T.E., and Whicker, F.W., 'Tissue distribution of radiocesium in the mule deer', *Health Physics* 1971, 21 (6), 862–6

Hiatt, G.S., 'Plutonium dispersal by mule deer at Rocky Flats, Colorado', MS thesis, Colorado State University, Fort Collins 1977

Joly, D.O., et al., 'Spatial epidemiology of chronic wasting disease in Wisconsin white-tailed deer', *J. Wildlife Diseases* 2006 July, 42 (3), 578–88

Little, C.A., 'Plutonium in a grassland ecosystem', PhD thesis, Colorado State University, Fort Collins, 1979

Purdey, M., 'High dose exposure to systemic phosmet insecticide modifies the phosphatidylinositol anchor on the prion protein; the origins of new variant transmissible spongiform encephalopathy?' *Med. Hypotheses* 1998, 50 (2), 91–111

Purdey, M., Ecosystems supporting clusters of sporadic TSEs demonstrate excesses of the radical generating divalent cation, manganese and deficiencies of antioxidant co-factors Cu, Se, Fe, Zn. Does a foreign cation substitution at Prp's Cu domain initiate TSE? *Med. Hypotheses* 2000, 54 (2), 278–306

Purdey, M., 'Elevated silver, barium and strontium in antlers, vegetation and soils sourced from CWD cluster areas: do Ag/Ba/Sr piezoelectric crystals represent the transmissible pathogenic agent in TSEs?' *Med. Hypotheses* 2004, 63 (2), 211–25

Spraker, T.R., Miller, M.W., Williams, E.S., Getzy, D.M., Adrian, W.J., Schoonveld, G.G., Spowart, R.A., O'Rourke, K.I., Miller, J.M., and Merz, P.A., 'Spongiform encephalopathy in free ranging mule deer, white-tailed deer and Rocky Mountain elk in north-central Colorado', *J. Wildlife Diseases* 1997, 33 (1), 1–6

Underhill, P.T., *Naturally Occurring Radioactive Material*, Advances in Environmental Series, St Lucie Press, Florida 1996

Whicker, F.W., Farris, G.C., Remmenga, E.E., and Dahl, A.H., 'Factors influencing the accumulation of fallout Cs 137 in Colorado mule deer', *Health Physics* 1965, 11, 1407–14

Whicker, F.W., Farris, G.C., and Dahl, A.H., 'Concentration patterns of Sr 90, Cs 137, I 131 in a wild deer population and environment', in Aberg, B., Hungate, F.P. (eds) *Radioecological Concentration Processes*, Pergamon Press, New York 1966, pp. 621–3

Williams, E.S., and Young, S., 'Chronic wasting disease of captive mule deer; a spongiform encephalopathy', *Journal of Wildlife Diseases* 1980, 16, 89–98

Chapter 7 The Road to Syracuse

Becker, R., and Selden, G., *The Body Electric*, Harper Paperbacks

Brown, P., et al., New studies on the heat resistance of hamster-adapted scrapie agent: threshold survival after ashing at 600 degrees C suggests an inorganic template of replication', *Proc. Natl. Acad. Sci.* 2000 Mar. 28, 97 (7), 3418–21

Gajdusek, D.C., 'Hypothesis: interference with axonal transport of neurofilament as a common pathogenetic mechanism in certain diseases of the CNS', *New England J. Med.* 1985, 312 (11), 714–18

Purdey, M., 'Metal microcrystal pollutants: the heat resistant, transmissible nucleating agents that initiate the pathogenesis of TSEs?' *Med. Hypotheses* 2005, 65 (3), 448–77

Purdey, M., 'Auburn University research substantiates the hypothesis that metal microcrystal nucleators initiate the pathogenesis of TSEs', *Med. Hypotheses* 2006, 66 (1), 197–9. Epub 13 Oct. 2005

Stanford, C.M., et al., 'Rapidly forming apatitic mineral in an osteoblastic cell line (UMR 106-01 BSP)', *J. Biol. Chem.* 1995 Apr. 21, 270 (16), 9420–8

Takeuchi, Y., et al., 'Isolation and characterization of proteoglycans synthesized by mouse osteoblastic cells in culture during the mineralization process', *Biochem. J.* 1990 Feb. 15, 266 (1), 15–24

Chapter 8 The Silicon Valleys

Purdey, M., 'Metal microcrystal pollutants: the heat resistant, transmissible nucleating agents that initiate the pathogenesis of TSEs?' *Med. Hypotheses* 2005, 65 (3) 448–77

Purdey, M., 'Auburn university research substantiates the hypothesis that metal microcrystal nucleators initiate the pathogenesis of TSEs'. *Med. Hypotheses* 2006, 66 (1), 197–9. Epub 13 Oct. 2005

Chapter 10 Behind the Iron Curtain

Bhattacharyya, S.D., and Sugiyama, H., 'Inactivation of botulinum and tetanus toxins by chelators', *Infect. Immun.* 1989, 57 (10), 3053–7

Cronje, L., and Bornman, L., 'Iron overload and tuberculosis; a case for iron chelation therapy', *Int. J. Tuberculosis and Lung Disease*, 2005 Sept. (1) 2–9

Flett, Sir J.S., Map of iron ores of England and Wales. Geological Survey of Great Britain; Ordnance Survey Office, Southampton 1935

Gobin, J., and Horwitz, M.A., 'Exochelins of mycobacterium tuberculosis remove iron from human iron-binding proteins and donate iron to mycobactins in the *M. tuberculosis* cell wall', *J. Experimental Med.* 1996, 183, 1527–32

Johnson-Ifearulundu, Y.J., and Kaneene, J.B., 'Relationship between soil type and mycobacterium paratuberculosis', *Am. Vet. Med. Ass.* 1997, 210, 1735–40

McDonald, P., Edwards, R.A., and Greenhalgh, J.F.D., *Animal Nutrition*, 2nd edn, Longman, London 1973

Pais, I., and Benton Jones, J., *The Handbook of Trace Elements*, St Lucie Press, Florida, 1997

Purdey, M., 'Anti-lactoferrin toxicity and elevated iron: the environmental pre-requisites which activate susceptibility to tuberculosis infection?' *Med. Hypotheses* 2006, 66 (3), 513–17. Epub 1 Dec. 2005

Ratledge, C., 'Iron, myobacteria and tuberculosis', *Tuberculosis* (Edin.) 2004, 84 (1–2), 110–30

Schaible, U.E., Collins, H.L., Priem, F., and Kaufmann, S.H., 'Correction of the iron overload defect in beta-2 microglobulin knockout mice by lactoferrin abolishes their increased susceptibility to tuberculosis', *J. Experimental Med.* 2002, 196 (11), 1507–13

Underwood, E.J., *Trace Elements in Human and Animal Nutrition*, 4th edn, Academic Press, London 1977

Weinberg, E., 'Iron loading and disease surveillance'. *Emerging Infectious Diseases*, 5 (3), 346–52

Afterword: Farewell

Chien-che Ying, Y. Fun-chang Wang, and Hanfen Tang, 'Icons of Medicinal Fungi from China' 1987

Csatary, L.K., Gosztonyk, G., Szeberenyi, J., Fabian, Z., Liszka, V., Bodey, B., and Csatary, C.M., 'TH-68/H oncolytic viral treatment in human high-grade gliomas',

J. Neurooncol., 2004 Mar.–Apr., 67 (1–2), 83–93. *Cancer Res.* 2005 Feb. 1, 65 (3), 999–1006

Chung, W.J., et al., 'Inhibition of cystine uptake disrupts the growth of primary brain tumors', *J. Neurosci.* 2005 Aug. 3, 25 (31), 7101–10

Kodama, N., et al. 'Can maitake MD-fraction aid cancer patients?' *Altern. Med. Rev.* 2002 June, 7 (3), 236–9. Review

Kuo, P.L., and Lin, C.C., 'Green tea constituent (-)-epigallocatechin-3-gallate inhibits Hep G2 cell proliferation and induces apoptosis through p53-dependent and Fas-mediated pathways'. *J. Biomed Sci.* 2003 Mar.–Apr., 10 (2), 219–27

Markert, J.M., et al., 'Oncolytic HSV-1 for the treatment of brain tumours', *Herpes* 2006 Nov., 13 (3), 66–71. Review

Nam, S.W., et al., 'Spontaneous regression of a large hepatocellular carcinoma with skull metastasis', *J. Gastroenterol. Hepatol.* 2005 Mar., 20 (3), 488–92 (*Phellinus linteus* treatment)

Ramos, S., et al., 'Comparative effects of food-derived polyphenols on the viability and apoptosis of a human hepatoma cell line (HepG2)', *J. Agric. Food Chem.* 2005 Feb. 23, 53 (4), 1271–80

Appendix: Don't let the buggers get you down

Anway, M.D., and Skinner, M.K., 'Epigenetic transgenerational actions of endocrine disruptors', *Endocrinology* 2006 June, 147 (6 Suppl.), S43–9. Epub 11 May 2006. Review

Behan, P.O., 'Chronic fatigue syndrome as a delayed reaction to chronic low-dose organophosphate exposure', *Journal of Nutritional and Environmental Medicine* 1996, 6 (4), 341–50

Behan, P.O., and Haniffah, B.A.G., 'Chronic fatigue syndrome: a possible delayed hazard of pesticide exposure' [Abstract], *Clinical Infectious Diseases* 1994; 18 (Supp. 1), S54

Brown, T.P., et al., 'Pesticides and Parkinson's disease – is there a link?' *Environmental Health Perspectives* 2006 Feb., 114 (2), 156–64

Carmine, A., et al., 'Further evidence for an association of the paraoxonase 1 (PON1) Met-54 allele with Parkinson's disease', *Mov. Disord.* 2002 July, 17 (4), 764–6

Cherry, N., et al., 'Paraoxonese (PON1) polymorphisms in farmers attributing ill health to sheep dip', *Lancet* 2002 Mar. 2, 359 (9308), 763–4

Compston, J.E., Vedi, S., Stephens, A.B., Bord, S., Lyons, A.R., Hodges, S.J., and Scammell, B.E., 'Reduced bone formation after exposure to organophosphates', *Lancet* 1999 Nov. 20, 354 (9192), 1791–2

Hope, J., and Baybutt, H., 'The key role of the nerve membrane protein PrP in scrapie-like diseases'. *Seminars in the Neurosciences*, Vol. 3, 1991, pp. 165–71

Jamal, G.A., Hansen, S., and Julu, P.O., 'Low level exposures to organophosphorus esters may cause neurotoxicity', *Toxicology* 2002 Dec. 27, 181–2, 23–33. Review

Jirtle, R.L., and Skinner, M.K., 'Environmental epigenomics and disease susceptibility', *Nat. Rev. Genet.* 2007 Apr., 8 (4), 253–62

Kamel, F., Hoppin, J.A., 'Association of pesticide exposure with neurologic dysfunction and disease', *Environmental Health Perspectives* 2004 June, 112 (9), 950–8

Mellick, G.D., 'CYP450, genetics and Parkinson's disease: gene × environment interactions hold the key', *J. Neural Transm. Suppl.* 2006 (70), 159–65

Menegon, A., et al., 'Parkinson's disease, pesticides, and glutathione transferase polymorphisms', *Lancet* 1998 Oct. 24, 352 (9137), 1344–6

Morahan, J.M., et al., 'Study of the paraoxonase 1 gene and pesticides in amyotrophic lateral sclerosis', *Neurotoxicology* 2006 Nov. 26

Newcombe, D.S., 'Immune surveillance, organosphosphorus exposure, and lymphomagenesis', *Lancet* 1992 Feb. 29, 339 (8792), 539–41

Pall, H.S., et al., 'Motoneurone disease as manifestation of pesticide toxicity', *Lancet* 1987 Sept. 19, 2 (8560), 685. No abstract available

Purdey, M., 'Mad cows and warble flies', *Ecologist* 1994, 24 (3) 100–4

Ray, D.E., and Richards, P.G., 'The potential for toxic effects of chronic, low-dose exposure to organophosphates', *Toxicol. Lett.* 2001 Mar. 31, 120 (1–3), 343–51. Review

Index